T0208258

CAN YOU LIVE FOREVER?

YOUR EXTENDED LIFE AND CONTINUED AWARENESS A SCIENTIFIC PERSPECTIVE

EDWARD W. REESE, Ph.D.

authorHOUSE

AuthorHouse™
1663 Liberty Drive
Bloomington, IN 47403
www.authorhouse.com
Phone: 833-262-8899

Published by AuthorHouse   03/02/2023

ISBN: 979-8-8230-0235-6 (sc)
ISBN: 979-8-8230-0234-9 (hc)
ISBN: 979-8-8230-0236-3 (e)

Library of Congress Control Number: 2023903731

Print information available on the last page.

This book is printed on acid-free paper.

contents

To my wife, Susan Beth, who has championed
my endeavors for over forty years

Acknowledgments

I thank my sister, Stella, and my brother-in-law, John Ey, for their continued support and encouragement with my professional and personal life issues.

Thank you to all the brilliant research scientists and a wide spectrum of authors for their knowledge and insights who have contributed to the contents of this book. Without their contribution, this book would not have been possible.

preface

Can Human Awareness Exist Forever?

Well, maybe the word *forever* is a little strong; however, based upon the direction and advancements in neuroscience, medicine, and other related fields discussed herein, there is, in my opinion, sufficient credible data and insights to recognize the possibility of greatly extended life well beyond the death of a normal life span. We will ponder this potential reality and explore the scientific pathway that may one day avail to humanity the possibility of extending human awareness into the realm of proportional, if not near-total, continued existence.

Also, if you are under thirty years of age, based upon current medical research findings, biomedical scientific advancements, and justified speculations discussed within this book, you will more likely than not, live to the age of one hundred and possibly longer, barring any intervening life hazard such as terminal illness or traumatic injury.

Important Clarification

I want to clarify up front that the entire contents of this reading is based on scientific fact or, at a minimum, justifiable scientific speculation. This includes all opinions I have offered regarding a multitude of related topics. Although some issues presented herein will certainly appear to be more in the realm of a science-fiction novel and difficult to accept as containing any acceptable reality, I assure you that as disconcerting and troubling as some opinions and predictions will appear, they are indeed believed to be accurate and strongly based upon the extrapolation of relevant scientific medical research and other contributing factors and are more likely to occur than not.

Read on …

Introduction

Your Extended Life and Continued Awareness

You are about to experience a discussion about topics that pertain to the extension of human life and the continued existence of human awareness. This writing will take you through an evolution of past and present accomplishments and future expectations, ultimately contributing to the extension of human life and continued awareness.

You should be informed that some aspects of this book are not for the light of heart and deals with subject matter that some may find troublesome and unsettling. Some parts are not PG-13 reading. In other words, "Reader discretion is advised." This acknowledgment is particularly relevant to the later sections of this writing and constitutes a smaller portion of this book.

However, having said that, be assured that all the material provided within this discussion is solidly based on truth, relevant facts, and scientifically-based speculation pertaining to future possibilities and expectations involving extended life and continued awareness, as interpreted and extrapolated from my review of scientifically-based, peer-reviewed articles, including my own extensive background dealing with much of the same subject matter.

What was once portrayed as pure science fiction now falls more into the realm of scientific fact or at least qualified scientific speculation regarding the more advanced thinking of extending life and awareness.

This book attempts to lay the historic foundation, current precepts, future speculations, and understanding that lends credence and justification for the journey toward and the ultimate arrival of a time in the foreseeable future when death is not a necessarily foregone conclusion, at least as pertains to your extended life and continued awareness. Indeed, I conclude it may not be necessary that your conscious awareness must inevitability surrender to an abnormality or failure of a vital body function or disease.

Moreover, this book is written for the average, everyday reader. It is not a text or intended for scientific review. It is very much intended to provide you with insights pertaining to the possible extension of your life and your continued awareness now and in the near and distant future.

Awareness and *life extension* are the predominant terms and ultimate focus throughout this book. I present my opinions, speculations, predictions, and conclusions on near and distant future expected scientific achievements toward life extension based upon my current interpretations of relevant advancements in medical science, applicable medical and bioengineering fields, and related industries that provide for our continued evolution from the earliest phase of inquiry to the furthest reaches of when we can anticipate that scientific research may ultimately take us regarding extending life and awareness.

To be specific, it is my opinion that life is most accurately defined as requiring awareness. If there is no awareness, then there is no life, understanding that the physical body can continue to exist by means of mechanical and other forms of life-supporting mechanisms and drugs required to artificially maintain the physical body, but absent conscious awareness. Life extension is the vehicle that could transport your awareness beyond your otherwise limited life span and even beyond the physical death of your body.

Based upon the exceptionally large number of complex and varied topics that should be addressed to accomplish a reasonable understanding of one's continued extended life and awareness would encompass a mammoth undertaking and formidable documentation. Therefore, visualize a wagon wheel with the hub representing the combined topics relevant to extended life and awareness, with each spoke contributing a particular scientific discipline to a consolidated but varied comprehension of these topics from the past and current understanding and as speculated for the near and distant future.

The formidable burden was to sift through these related but different scientific research studies and other contributing variables and to separate and consolidate the more focused material that would enhance and clarify a better understanding of this investigation for your consideration.

You will obviously note there is quite often no harmonious relationship or consensus of agreement between the various key players (e.g., scientists, futurists, health-care providers, religious and ethics groups, governing agencies, etc.) pertaining to the most appropriate direction, if any, toward extending life based upon their individual area of belief, expertise, and responsibility.

As you ponder the sensibility of the subject matter that follows, please remember that within the realm of scientific inquiry and the search for discovery and truth, it is particularly prudent to understand that the term never should never be used. In those circumstances where it is tempting for scientists to conclude that such-and-such could never occur, the door upon such conclusions must remain open a crack to future discovery possibilities. History has demonstrated that what was once considered impossible has often evolved to become a reality in the future.

I have attempted to provide a fair appraisal and presentation for both sides as viewed by those who believe strongly in the possibility of these highly controversial topics as well as those who strongly disagree and other conflicting opinions in between.

While recognizing that these scientists and other contributors are highly qualified with extensive experience and qualifications within their individual but related occupations, I have assumed the position of (hopefully) unbiased observer (to a practical extent) to balance these controversial subjects and present to you what, in my opinion, represents a middle-of-the-road position relevant to the subject topics.

As a forensic examiner, investigator, and research scientist for over thirty-four years, I have investigated many hundreds of cases attempting to determine the cause(s) and contributing factors to a patient's serious injury or death. To successfully accomplish this task, I have refined my methodology of investigation to first gathering as much relevant evidence and details as possible. Only after a thorough investigation would I produce my concluding opinions to present at deposition and in both state and federal courts wherein I have been approved by the courts as an expert in these related fields of medicine and scientific research and qualified to submit my concluding opinions.

I have also applied my validated methods of investigating the evidence and details presented throughout this discussion by the various scientists, futurists, and other relevant participants in order to reach an acceptable threshold determination, within the realm of my purview, as to what is the most prudent, logical, and realistic conclusions to the subject matter at hand.

My opinions and observations should encourage you to consider both sides of the opinion coin and to ferret out which controversial side of the topic you believe is more in keeping with your own thinking. I encourage you to apply your own independent analysis and considerations to the many controversial topics presented within this reading. Moreover, consider why you formulated your particular conclusions. Can you identify any historic experience that influenced you to a particular bias?

Each major contributing participant whose published research findings or discussions pertaining to extended life and awareness has remained steadfast in their opinions with no apparent desire for synergistic collaboration, especially with other scientists who maintain opposing opinions.

However, I have interjected my opinions and conclusions, as I trust you will do the same, after evaluating the data, commentary, discussion, and justification provided by both sides regarding the extension of one's life and awareness. An example of the controversy follows.

There are those who oppose attempts at life extension for various reasons. For example, Leon Kass, chairman of the U.S. President's Council on Bioethics, has voiced his concern that extending the life of a population would result in overpopulation problems and therefore would be unethical.[1] The subject of overpopulation resulting from the successful extension of human life is discussed in greater detail later in this reading.

Kass has further stated,

> Simply to covet a prolonged life span for ourselves is both a sign and a cause of our failure to open ourselves to procreation (reproduce) and to any higher purpose. The desire to prolong youthfulness is not only a childish desire to eat one's life and keep it; it is also an expression of a childish and narcissistic wish incompatible with devotion to posterity.[2]

However, many others, including myself, hold the same opinion as John Harris, former editor-in-chief of the *Journal of Medical Ethics*, "as long as life is worth living, according to the person himself, we have a powerful moral imperative to save life and thus to develop and offer life extension therapies to those who want them."[3]

Controversy about life extension is due, in part, to fears of overpopulation and possible effects on society. Gerontologist Aubrey De Grey counters the overpopulation critique by pointing out, "The therapy could postpone or eliminate menopause, allowing women to space out their pregnancies over more years and thus decreasing the yearly population growth."[4]

Some philosophers and futurists like Max More erroneously believe, in my opinion, that the worldwide population is slowing down and will eventually stabilize and even decrease; therefore,

---

[1] "Life extension," en.wikipedia.org/wiki/Life extension.
[2] Id.
[3] Id.
[4] Id.

extended longevity would not contribute to overpopulation.[5] Quite to the contrary, historic and current data clearly indicates a continued and ever-increasing population worldwide. In fact, the numbers are staggering and should cause one to pause and contemplate a dismal future for humanity.

Reviewing the historical struggle to exist and evolve over the centuries by humans can be visualized as initially climbing a steep hill that becomes less steep with the passing of time due to medical and scientific advancements that have extended life and reduced or eliminated associated pain and suffering, both physically and psychologically. Goals within these fields have become easier to reach and further facilitate continued progress by building upon a better understanding of these issues from prior and current achievements and discovery.

However, the contents of this review include supportive data and details that in themselves are highly controversial, pertaining to the extension of life, opinions, speculations, and conclusions by medical research scientists, health-care providers, religious groups, the medical and pharmaceutical industry, Food and Drug Administration (FDA), legal community, and others.

Therefore, the spectrum of agreeing with or rejecting the opinions, conclusions, or speculations from either side of the relevant issues of this writing is ultimately left to your interpretation and judgment since the disparities are often quite significant and diverse.

Nonetheless, this book attempts to establish and present a viable and plausible foundation focused upon each of the key variable topics that should be considered in formulating your own conclusions about the various evolutionary stages of life extension and awareness.

A significant attempt has been made to provide current and historic thinking by qualified and reputable professionals within each of their related fields and on both sides of the topic, but only to the minimal extent estimated to be (hopefully) sufficient for an adequate understanding of the subject matter as presented by these scientists.

---

[5] Id.

Since there is such a diverse level of acceptance, rejection, and understanding or interpretation as to the many contributing factors associated with the focus and topics of extending life and awareness, I have defined many of the relevant terms in order to establish a more concise, focused, and consolidated understanding of these significant issues.

The critical individual intervening variables involve different subject matter pertaining to extending life, which have been discussed and argued about for many years, is more controversial now than ever before. The applicable issues that must be explored and amalgamated before passing judgment along the spectrum of your acceptance or rejection involves many other significant considerations, criteria, and variables, including ethics, morals, religious beliefs, unknowns, and so forth that individually would present their respective spectrum of concepts, justifications, understanding, and forethought.

While reading this book, you should develop an appreciation and hopefully a better understanding of the incredible functions of the human brain and its many abilities. You should also formulate your own value judgments and levels of acceptance or rejection based on the uniqueness and idiosyncrasies of who you are and how you process the subject matter.

It is my concluding opinion that ultimately our continued existence (our awareness) will not be dependent upon the function of the human physical body, which in many respects presents a hindrance to our continued existence beyond our current estimated life span. There are simply too many body components that we must depend upon to function effectively to maintain our lives and awareness to continue. The vulnerability of critical organs, too many diseases, and failures most often cause premature termination of the body and subsequently the demise of a healthy brain and awareness.

Your assessment of each major topic and its contributing factors to extending life and awareness may prove challenging. Your self-appraisal of these subjects will have been formulated, in part, based upon your own personal life experiences that ultimately established your individual beliefs, perspectives, and opinions, as influenced by your parental relationships, education, religion, friends, and other influencing factors starting at a young age.

Thus, you have developed opinions and assigned values to your precepts that vary and change over time as you subconsciously process and amalgamate your evolving life experiences. Some of your life's experiences may have been traumatic, resulting in you forming some strong negative opinions on certain life issues. Conversely, you most likely experienced some positive remembrance that formed loving and endearing feelings for others and subjects that bring you joy and comfort.

Which topics tend to influence you the most in either a positive or negative manner? Is there a point in your thinking where medical research has progressed too far, especially when the existence of what is considered normal physical, anatomical, and physiological aspects of life and awareness have advanced to artificial methods required to extend life and consciousness?

You may find it interesting and insightful to have your family members and friends review the subject matter of this book and then meet to discuss your individual opinions and conclusions and how each participant justifies their position. How rigid would you and the others hold to the individual perceptions and beliefs? What are the sticking points? At what point will you or another acknowledge, "That's as far as I am willing to go"? I am confident that you will discover some aspects to be very controversial and different among your family members and friends.

In progressing toward the hot topic issues that pertain to life extension and awareness, I will also discuss relevant and applicable issues dealing with the aging process and its relationship to extended life.

1
what is the ultimate question?

The ultimate question for extended life expectancy and thus our awareness is, "Why must my awareness cease to exist because a vital body organ fails or I have a terminal illness?" More specifically, "Why should my awareness with a healthy brain, cognizant of my life existence and my surroundings, cease to exist for reasons independent of any neurological causation but due to a body organ failure or disease?"

That's a darn-good question. The medical research attempting to answer that question is more driven now than at any prior time. The more progress and success in answering at least some portion of this critical and very relevant question for all humanity, the more science is motivated to press forward.

Awareness is life, and without the brain's capacity to accomplish a cognitive understanding of one's existence or obtain knowledge and interact within the environment, there is no viable life function; there is mere existence at best. The function of the brain is to produce awareness so we can effectively interact with others and respond to the circumstances of our surroundings appropriately. It allows us to experience and respond to the precepts, circumstances, and interpretations of daily life.

Rene Descartes, a seventeenth-century French philosopher, conducted a search for a statement that could not be doubted. Upon

1

concluding his search, Descartes coined the phrase in his *Discourse on Method* (1637), "I think, therefore I am." He found that he could not doubt his own existence and recognized that thinking does occur.[6] Therefore, Descartes's conclusion represents a direct link to the understanding of human awareness, the focus of this inquiry. Thinking is the process initiated from our awareness, and our awareness is governed by the incredible processing ability of our brains to formulate decisions and initiate our perceived and appropriate actions or reactions.

The Evolving Process to Extend Life

Since early civilization, and especially during the ages of the Roman and Greek empires, humankind has pondered their existence and their mortality, desiring a greater length of life and wondering how to extend their existence. With the passage of ages, life has continued to extend longer and longer to the present day. The brilliance of our time is getting closer than ever to discoveries that will eventually extend the length of life significantly.

Every six years, the average life span in the United States increases by another year. According to the 2010 U.S. Census, nearly one in seven Americans are sixty-five or older. By 2050, the Bureau estimates that this number will rise to more than one in five. Another sign of our increasing longevity is the growing number of people living well into old age. Between 1990 and 2009, the number of centenarians in the United States nearly tripled, from 38,300 to 104,099. By the middle of this century, the Bureau predicts that more than 400,000 people in the United States will be at least one hundred years old.[7]

Scientists have acquired a far greater understanding of why and how we age. For the first time in human history, scientists are now

---

[6] C. Miceli, "I Think Therefore I Am: Descartes on the Foundations of Knowledge," In *Word Philosophy – An Introductory Anthology* (2018), 2.
[7] M. Masci, "To Count Our Days: The Scientific and Ethical Dimensions of Radical Life Extension," https://www.pewresearch.org/experts/david-masci.

working with confidence on research projects that will eventually and dramatically extend the life of humankind. No longer is the horizon of our longevity limited to our traditional life spans. Research scientists now position themselves at the pinnacle of scientific discovery at the far end of traditional life limitations and push open the door to a new realm of longevity possibilities.

Although many research objectives have yet to disclose answers to the elusive secrets of extending life far beyond its current limitations, scientists continue to build upon their knowledge and insights previously gained with tantalizing clues to extending longevity further and further. Nonetheless, critical discoveries present a daunting and formidable challenge to finding solutions to obstacles that have yet to be overcome.

The contents of this inquiry, with its speculative but warranted predictions, opinions, and conclusions, are based upon and justified by a review of the historic and unabated constant evolution of medical science, advancements in medical technology and drugs, increased capabilities of the health-care provider, and a greater understanding of factors that cause or contribute to extending human life.

The anatomical and physiological structure of the human body is a wondrous and complex network composed primarily of cells, tissues, organs, and systems. There are eleven distinct organ systems in human beings, which form the basis of human anatomy and physiology, including the respiratory system, digestive and excretory system, circulatory system, urinary system, integumentary (skin) system, skeletal system, muscular system, endocrine system, lymphatic system, nervous system, and reproductive system.[8]

Every year, new advances and discoveries involving medical science and evolving medical products and pharmaceuticals are released into commercial distribution by the FDA. With each new technological advancement evolving from scientific research and product development, more innovative and advanced resources establish a broader foundation upon which future scientific

---

[8] "Organ system," en.wikipedia.org/wiki/Organ system.

discoveries will yield new medical products, drugs, and methods that further reduce pain and suffering.

Similar to the first flight by a primitive-powered aircraft on December 17, 1903, by the Wright brothers at Kitty Hawk, the advancements in flight technology have ultimately reached levels of supersonic aircraft, guided missiles, and spacecraft capable of reaching the moon and other planets. Henry Ford, an American industrialist, established the Ford Motor Company in 1903 and produced the first automobile, the Model T, in 1908.[9] Now we have advanced to high-performance vehicles, like the Lamborghini and Ferrari. In a comparative manner, the exponential advancements within the medical profession, academic pursuits, and medical industry have extended and enhanced life.

Aubrey de Grey, a former Cambridge University researcher and chief science officer at an antiaging think tank in Mountain View, California, believes aging will be conquered through a variety of rejuvenation biotechnologies that will repair and maintain the body indefinitely. Under this scenario, various treatments, including stem cell and gene therapies, would be applied at the cellular level to halt the damage to the body caused by aging. de Grey has stated during a 2011 interview that he believes there is a fifty-fifty chance of bringing the aging process under medical control within the next twenty-five years or so.[10]

Disconcerting, however, is the obvious reality that those who will initially benefit from new medical innovations that extend life will be the wealthy individuals who can afford the high cost of such life-extending technology and treatments. Therefore, such inevitable social disparities would eventually surface with the recognition that the haves in life will have even more, especially as pertaining to them living longer and gaining more wealth. Such inequalities and

---

[9] "Henry Ford," en.Wikipedia.org/wiki/Henry Ford.

[10] A. de Grey, "To Count Our Days: The Scientific and Ethical Dimension of Radical Life Extension," In "Who Wants to Live Forever? Scientist sees aging cured," http://www.reuters.com/article/2011/07/04/us-aging:cure-idUSTRE76321D20110704.

injustices may promote future social upheaval, as the life-extending benefits to the wealthy will produce a wider and wider gap.

Eventually, many of the life-extending treatments will become available to a larger population, but not everyone. Insurance companies will most likely not provide coverage or provide minimal coverage for such treatments based upon the procedures being determined to be elective and not related to maintaining the existing health of the individual.

However, it is not anticipated that the U.S. government would intervene with laws and regulations to prevent the life-extending treatments afforded only to the rich. They would not deny the wealthy access to such treatments just because they are not available to a much larger segment of the population. So what's new?

Moreover, the governing decision-makers may further reason that if life-extending treatments were made available to everyone, a far greater burden would affect overall living conditions due to significant overpopulation. Overpopulation becomes a topic of concern discussed in greater detail later.

What Do So Many Want So Desperately to Avoid?

What many people want so desperately to avoid is death. More specifically, they do not want to lose their self-awareness and the awareness of their environment, the activities taking place around them, and especially the awareness of their continued existence.

Death anxiety is anxiety caused by thoughts of one's own death and is also referred to as *thanatophobia*, meaning a fear of death.[11] Existential, pertaining to or dealing with existence,[12] death anxiety stems from the basic knowledge that human life must end. Existential death anxiety is known to be the most powerful form of death anxiety.[13]

---

[11] "Death Anxiety (psychology)," en.wikipedia.org/wiki/Death Anxiety.
[12] "Existential." The American Heritage Dictionary, Second College Edition.
[13] "Death Anxiety (psychology)," en.wikipedia.org/wiki/Death Anxiety.

5

It is the great unknown of death that many people fear and the knowledge that there isn't anything they can do about it. As time passes, these individuals who suffer from death anxiety become increasingly desperate with their situations and inability to reconcile an acceptance of the inevitable end of their existence (awareness).

Thus, many individuals waste significant portions of their lives worrying, often deeply, about their future death and when it might occur. These troubled individuals have such an intense fear of death that they may develop an innate belief that death may somehow be avoided and thus desperately spend a portion of their lives seeking out any potential resource that could conceivably provide them with a way to avoid death, usually within the domain of the occult, some other paranormal group, or fraudulent medical products or drugs.

These individuals, and others who are not quite as desperate and wealthy, would look favorably upon potential options to avoid death by putting down a deposit for such radical and unproven procedures, such as cryogenic cold storage of their body, head, or brain, as discussed later.

Such fearful people would also consider any future options that offers the potential to extend their continued awareness, including brain, head, and body transplants and awareness transfers if and when they would be made available. These individuals are also typically hypochondriacs who constantly run to their physician or hospital, believing that any pain may produce a serious injury or even death.

Conversely, many other religious followers, like Christians, believe the person's awareness does not cease to exist after their death, but rather moves on to a continuing awareness of their existence and into a much happier realm (e.g., heaven) after their death.

There are, generally speaking, two sides of the coin to consider when asking the question, "What is it that so many want so desperately to avoid?" Psychologists, neurologists, and other related fields of scientific study would conclude that such limitations are far too narrow to properly answer the question. However, for my purposes, I only want to state the obvious without going too far afield on the subject. Therefore, on the one side is the fear, sometimes overwhelming fear of death, or death anxiety. At the extreme, these people are gripped in a continual fear of dying so intense that their daily life is often incapacitated by their hampered inability to live a normal life.

More typical of those who would answer, "Yes, I do fear dying and death," are those who would begrudgingly acquiesce to the reality that there isn't anything they can do about avoiding the inevitable encroachment of their demise and continue with their daily living, although with less trepidation than those who process their eventual death almost daily.

On the other side, a lot of interest and debate surrounds the question of what happens to one's conscious mind (awareness) as the body dies. According to some neuroscientific views that see these processes as the physical basis of a mental phenomenon, the mind fails to survive brain death and ceases to exist. This permanent loss of consciousness and awareness after death is sometimes called "eternal oblivion." The belief by others that some spiritual or incorporeal component (soul) exists and is preserved after death is described by the term *afterlife*.[14]

Thus, there are two primary beliefs as to the afterlife existence, one based upon most scientific thinking that after death, there is only "eternal oblivion" (i.e., no so-called afterlife awareness, nothing). In my opinion, such conclusions would certainly produce a dismal, depressing, and discouraging sense of existence, believing that one's current existence is all that there is.

As a research investigator myself, I prefer the second conclusion that there is indeed an awareness that continues after this life experience, primarily based on my faith. While many believe it is foolish to anticipate a conscious awareness in an afterlife, more and more scientists are leaving the door open a crack on the subject primarily due, in part, to the large number of individuals from all walks of life who have had a dramatic change of opinion after they

---

[14] "Mind," en.wikipedia.org/wiki/Mind.

personally had a near-death experience (NDE), an awareness of their existence after an apparent life-ending tragedy.

For example, there have been many such events reported where a patient has died during surgery (flatlined) on the table and subsequently awakened (returned from momentary death) and described hovering over their body and observing the surgical procedure, the instruments being used, the surgical team, and even the discussion of the staff while they were determined to be clinically dead.

Otherwise, I find it difficult and unsettling to conclude that we exist for a very finite period of time, some for only a few years, and then disappear into nothing. That would seem so pointless, but there it is, a matter of faith or science, no condemnation intended to those who dedicate themselves to scientific endeavors, as I do as well, just different concluding realties.

For many thousands, the question of a possible afterlife existence has been answered, and for these individuals, there is no doubt about what awaits them after death. Again, I am referring to the NDE. These survivors are convinced that an afterlife existence does in fact await them, and many of them are actually looking forward to returning to what they experienced during the time they were determined to be clinically dead. They come from all walks of life and include a spectrum of personal and professional backgrounds, including physicians, scientists, college professors, and those with very little education to those with distinguished academic credentials.

Most individuals who have reported the phenomenon of a NDE have very similar experiences, including an overwhelming sense of peace and well-being, detachment from their physical body, levitation, and ability to hover over the location of their death episode and hear and visually describe the events taking place during their out-of-body existence.

They also experience absolute freedom from all burdens, witness a meeting with a departed loved ones, encounter more friends and family members who had passed on, and observe the presence of a light, sometimes within a tunnel. The sum total of their NDE produces a strong desire to remain where they were during their afterlife time and not to return to their physical body or their prior existence. After returning to their body and awakening to the reality of the person they were prior to their afterlife experience, almost all describe a profound change to their personal character, their attitude about life, and the belief that there is a continued awareness involving a heavenly existence after life has ended.

It is particularly interesting and insightful to listen to professional, highly educated technical and scientific individuals, including those with medical research backgrounds and physicians, who themselves had a NDE. Many had the opinion and were often adamant before their out-of-body revelation into an apparent afterlife existence that there is no existence, no awareness after death, and even offered apparent scientific evidence to support their alleged conclusions. Most were somewhat sheepish in their post-afterlife experience to reconcile their dramatic life-changing revelation with their prior belief that what they experience could not occur. Subsequently, most, if not all, concluded they could not explain what they had experienced.

What Is Life?

There are so many definitions of life based on various religious beliefs, cultures, and superstitions that it would be impractical to cite just one or two definitions as fully representative of the term. However, I believe the following basic definitions are uniformly accepted.

Life is the interval of time between birth and death and the time period for which humans exists or functions. However, for the purpose of this analysis, this definition will not suffice. Thus, life is further defined as follows:

> The most essential understanding of the term *life* is the imposed term *awareness* as a critical neurological and cognitive function in understanding the meaning and value of life and the ability to extend and comprehend life with a prerequisite criteria and expectation of

continued awareness. Therefore, awareness is life and without awareness there is no life.

But let's take this a step further. Since scientists started taking a serious look at extending the life of humanity beyond the standard limits of a normal life cycle, as is the focus of this discussion, they have been placing less and less dependency upon the body to support their efforts. That certainly sounds like a contradiction of terms; however, I am referring to the extension of life, meaning awareness, beyond the limits imposed upon awareness by the functions of the body and its vulnerable parts.

Now without losing focus on the definition of life, what aspect of the total human body constitutes human life? In other words, what are the prerequisites for a human body to have life? It may not be as black-and-white as you may think, and the consequences of attempting to define life will become more problematic as scientists venture further into the evolutionary progression of their efforts to extend human existence.

Stay with me. In other words, as we develop an appreciation as to where the bioscience, neuroscience, and other related scientific endeavors are leading us regarding future brain and head transplants and awareness transfers into artificial brains, how do we continue to define human life? Where does life actually reside? Is it the functioning of the heart, the brain, or any other vital organ(s)? For example, if the brain or the head were transplanted to another body, would that represent a transfer of life to the donor's body? There presumedly would be life if our definition of life requiring awareness held true. But hold on.

If so, then how do we reconcile the body of the donor's corpse, which at the point of transplantation is assumed to have been resurrected back to a living entity? Otherwise, the transfer of awareness would not be effective. This dilemma is further discussed from a different perspective starting in chapter 10.

Confusing, I know; however, these two terms, *life* and *awareness*, will walk hand in hand for a limited period. Eventually awareness will let go of the hand of life since any vestige of a shared relationship will no longer exist. There will come a time in the distant future when the transfer of human awareness will be so complete and independent of the body (e.g., life) that the term *awareness* can no longer be defined as including human life.

What Is Death, and When Does It Occur?

There is limitless conjecture and debate over what occurs to our awareness or consciousness once the physical body has been declared legally dead. Legally dead is determined today by a qualified physician or health-care provider with proper training who has deemed that the individual has no respiration (breathing), heart rate, or brain activity, including the brain stem.

There are three primary causes of death: aging, disease, and body trauma. For hundreds of years, two primary aspects of death have been debated:

1. Initially, only a rudimentary concern to determine if a person were alive or dead was relevant. However, many times this obvious determination was inaccurate, as most of us have read or heard of individuals who woke up buried in a dark coffin to discover the unimaginable horror of their circumstance. Based upon the few bodies that have been exhumed and subsequently discovered damage to the interior of the coffin by the revived body, one can only speculate as to how many others experienced such an indescribable and horrific experience. Moreover, there have been many more individuals who have been reported to awaken in the coroner's facility or a funeral home prior to embalming.

   While the methods of determining actual death have not always been accurate or professionally determined over the years, a far more definitive protocol has been established, and a more accurate assessment of when physical death has occurred is currently universally accepted, as described previously.

11

Currently, the most definitive method of determining a person's death is the threshold assessment of brain death, meaning that all brain functions have permanently ceased.

2. The second criteria of death is the actual and accurate time of death. For hundreds of years, there was little attention or focus applied to determining the time a person died. However, with the dramatic advancements in medicine and science, it is now critical to know the closest estimate to the time of actual death, especially pertaining to organ transplantation. It is life dependent that a donor's organ is properly transferred to the recipient's hospital as quickly as possible. Due to the critical nature and viability of the donor's body to prove appropriate for the intended recipient, the standard of body acceptance is now dependent upon very precisely defined criteria.

In the United States and many other countries, a person is legally dead if they permanently lose all brain activity (brain death) or all breathing and circulatory functions.[15] Brain stem death is the standard of death in the UK and entails that death has occurred if the brain stem alone, as opposed to the whole brain, has ceased to function.[16]

I will not belabor the discussion about death any further than indicated previously. It is only mentioned in that the focus of this book is upon extending one's life and conscience awareness beyond the time of anticipated death or immediately thereafter. However, I will offer one related and interesting concept about death, as described by Aubrey de Grey, a prior Cambridge University researcher and chief science officer at an anti-aging think tank in Mountain View, California.

de Grey's group, the Strategies for Engineered Negligible Senescence (SENS) Research Foundation, says that people fear much

---

[15] R. Rettner, "Life After Brain Death: Is the Body Still Alive?" Live Science.
[16] G. Schofield et al., "When does a human being die? Brain Stem Death," *QJM: An International Journal of Medicine* 108 (2014), 605–609. https://doi.org/10.1093/qjmed/hcu239.

longer life spans only because they have been persuaded to believe that death is natural and even good. de Grey refers to this form of thinking as a "pro-aging trance," which he says was a sensible way of coping with the inevitability of aging when it was inevitable. But now that aging and dying might not be inevitable, this mindset has become part of the problem.[17]

It is not natural and not part of our genetic awareness to view death as a good thing. The entire process and exhaustive efforts of brilliant scientists and research institutions have dedicated their combined pursuits and professional careers, both individually and as a consolidated effort, to extend life because extended life provides a positive benefit to both the individual and humankind.

To accept the inevitability of death as a natural and good thing defeats the committed efforts and goals to defeat its finality, in part or in whole. This is certainly not to suggest that death is not a reality today, as indeed those of us alive today are condemned to our ultimate demise.

Nonetheless, today we can ponder the tantalizing prospects of a radical life extension as realistic and plausible. Its eventuality is like looking at a blurry movie screen that becomes clearer and more recognizable with the passage of time. Currently, regarding radical life extension, we are looking at a blurry screen, but at a minimum, we are now looking at the screen that will eventually gain greater clarity and thereby provide increasing hope and excitement for future accomplishments.

Annual Leading Causes of Death in the United States

- Heart disease: 659,041
- Cancer: 599,601
- Accidents (unintentional injuries): 173,040
- Chronic lower respiratory disease: 156,979

---

[17] A. de Grey. "To Count Our Days: The Scientific and Ethical Dimensions of Radical Life Extension," In "Why We Age and How We Can Avoid It,http://www.youtube.com/watch?

EDWARD W. REESE, PH.D.

- Stroke (cerebrovascular disease): 150,005
- Alzheimer's disease: 121,499
- Diabetes: 87,647
- Nephritis, nephrotic syndrome, and nephrosis: 51,565
- Influenza and pneumonia: 49,783
- Intentional self-harm (suicide): 47,511[18]

The number-one cause of death in the United States pertains to the cardiovascular system. The most common change in the cardiovascular system is the stiffening of the blood vessels and arteries, causing your heart to work harder to pump blood through them. You can do the following to improve your cardiovascular system:

- Include physical activity in your daily routine.
- Eat a healthy diet.
- Don't smoke.
- Manage stress.
- Get enough sleep.[19]

Of course, as individuals commit themselves to fighting the various aging factors, their success will also extend their lives in keeping with the advancements of medical and neuroscientist endeavors to combat the aging process and further extend their lives.

---

[18] M. Kochanek, "Leading Causes of Death," Mortality in the United States, NCHS Data Brief No. 395.

[19] P.D. Takahashi, "Healthy Aging. Your Cardiovascular System," Mayo Clinic.

2

The Brain

Since the brain is the ultimate focus of this review, meaning that our continued existence and awareness is based upon the effective continuation of the brain function after the physical body has died, let's first discuss some of the more relevant and interesting aspects of the brain.

First, let's clarify some long-standing myths about the brain. One myth claims that humans only use a small percentage of its full potential or capability, for example, 10 percent. However, this is inaccurate. Brain scans have shown that we use pretty much all of our brains all of the time, even when we're asleep.[20]

Another common myth involves the belief that you predominantly use your left or your right brain. Once again, however, this is not true. While it is true that each of our hemispheres has slightly different roles, individuals do not actually have a dominant brain side that governs their personality and abilities. Instead, research has revealed that people use both brain hemispheres pretty much in equal measure.[21]

As humans age, their brains start to shrink, to lose neurons and the cognitive process, including memory formation and diminished

---

[20] M. Cohut, "Seven (or more) things you didn't know about your brain," https://www.medicalnewstoday.com/articles/322081#7.-Is-perception-a-controlled-hallucination?
[21] Id.

Edward W. Reese, Ph.D.

ability to recall memory. These functions start shrinking when we reach our sixties and seventies.[22]

Behavioral Brain Changes Over Human Life Span

Age Range	Behavioral Changes
Early Childhood	The foundation for lifelong brain function, memory, and adaptability
Preschool	is established/grows. Complex actions become possible (e.g., raising head, reaching, rolling, crawling, walking, and running).
School-Aged	The ability to understand, process, and respond to social situations increases.
Childhood	Between five to eleven years of age, many language and cognition milestones are reached.
Adolescence	The ability to reason about abstract concepts develops. Emotions are heightened in intensity and urgency.
Young Adulthood	Impulse control and planning abilities are mastered.
Middle Ages	Abstract reasoning, mathematical, and spatial (e.g., having the nature of space) reasoning and verbal abilities increase. Optimism and social appropriateness increase.
Older Ages	Complex mental processes may be negatively affected. Vocabulary and experience-based knowledge remain strengths. Speed of processing decreases, and extra time to complete tasks may be obvious.[23]

The human brain functions as the control center of the human nervous system. The brain stem connects the brain to the spinal cord, which then relays information to the body and back to the brain. Both the brain and spinal cord make up the central nervous system.

---

[22] Id.

[23] T. O'Neil-Pirozzi, "Traumatic Brain Injury Resource for Survivors and Caregivers," https://bouve.northeastern.edu/nutraumaticbraininjurybi-anatomy/brain-changes-over-the-lifespan.

A human adult brain weighs about three pounds and is approximately fifteen centimeters long. For comparison, a newborn baby's brain weights about three-quarters of a pound.[24]

Also consider the following:

- Your brain is not fully formed until age twenty-five.
- Brain information travels up to an impressive 268 miles per hour.
- A piece of brain tissue the size of a grain of sand contains 100,000 neurons and a billion synapses.
- The human brain can generate about 23 watts of power (enough to power a lightbulb).[25]
- The average male has a brain volume of 1,274 cubic centimeters.
- The average female brain has a volume of 1,131 cubic centimeters.
- The cerebrum contains about 86 billion nerve cells (neurons), the gray matter. It also contains billions of nerve fibers (axons and dendrites), the white matter.[26]

Some other interesting facts about the brain:

- **Multitasking is impossible.** When we think we're multitasking, we're actually context-switching. That is, we're quickly switching back and forth between different tasks rather than doing them at the same time. Research has determined that when you multitask, your error rate goes up 50 percent and it takes twice as long to do things.
- **Water makes up about 75 percent of the brain.** This means that dehydration, even as small as 2 percent, can have a

---

[24] K. Cherry, "The Size of the Human Brain," https://www.very wellmind.com/how-big-is-the-brain-2794888#:-:text=many other mammals.

[25] K. Sachdeva, "11 Fun Facts About Your Brain," https://www.nm.org/healthbeat/healthy-tips/11-fun-facts-about-your-brain.

[26] T. Lewis, "Human Brains: Facts, Functions & Anatomy," https://www.livescience.com/29365-human-brain.html.

negative effect on brain functions. Dehydration and a loss of sodium and electrolytes can cause acute changes in memory and attention.

- **Cholesterol is key to learning and memory.** The brain has a higher cholesterol content than any other organ. In fact, about 25 percent of the body's cholesterol resides within the brain. The brain is highly dependent on cholesterol. It produces its own cholesterol, which is more stable than the cholesterol in other organs.

- **A brain freeze is really a warning signal.** A brain freeze happens when you eat or drink something that's too cold. It chills the blood vessels and arteries in the very back of the throat, including the ones that take blood to your brain. These constrict when they're cold and open back up when they're warm again, causing the pain in your forehead. This is your brain telling you to stop what you are doing to prevent unwanted changes due to temperature.

- **The brain can't feel pain.** There are no pain receptors in the brain itself. Surgery can be done on the brain, and technically the brain does not feel that pain.

- **Your brain is a random thought generator.** In 2005, the National Science Foundation published an article regarding research about human thoughts per day. The average person has about 12,000 to 60,000 thoughts per day. Of those, 95 percent are exactly the same repetitive thoughts as the day before, and about 80 percent are negative.

- **Your brain uses 20 percent of the oxygen and blood in your body.** Your brain needs a constant supply of oxygen. As little as five minutes without oxygen can cause some brain cells to die, leading to severe brain damage. Also, the harder you think, the more oxygen and fuel your brain will use from your blood, up to 50 percent.

- **Reading out loud uses different brain circuits than reading silently.** Reading aloud promotes brain development. Children first learn to read by speaking words out loud.

Once that knowledge is established, then they learn to read to themselves. It's indeed one of the strange facts about the brain because we usually teach our children to read and talk politely. But to promote brain development in your child, you should read and talk aloud in front of them.

- **Your brain is mostly fat.** Consisting of a minimum of 60 percent fat, your brain is the fattiest organ in your body. This is why healthy fats, such as omega-3s and omega-6s, are vital for brain and overall body health. Healthy fat helps stabilize the cell walls in the brain. It can also reduce inflammation and help the immune system function properly.
- **Sleep is imperative.** Your body and brain require rest in order to function properly. Judgment, memory, and reaction time can all be impaired when someone does not have enough sleep. Sleep deprivation kills brain cells. Proper sleep is also essential for memory retention. During sleep, the brain accumulates all the memories from the day. Yawning cools down the brain. Sleep deprivation raises brain temperature.[27], [28]

Some neuroscientists now believe that many of our memories do not reside in the brain alone but represent combined memories. They believe that a post-op head transplant recipient would lose some of their prior memories and possibly gain some memories retained within the donor's body.

The Brain vs. the Mind

Brain and mind are not the same. Your brain is part of the visible, tangible world of the body. Your mind is part of the invisible, transcendent world of thought, feeling, attitude, belief, and imagination. The brain is the physical organ most associated with mind and consciousness, but the mind is not confined to the brain.

---

[27] D. Alban, "22 Facts About the Brain," bebrainfit.com/human-brain-facts.
[28] Id.

The intelligence of your mind permeates every cell of your body and has tremendous power over all bodily systems.[29]

The brain is the physical place where the mind resides. The mind is the manifestation of thought, perception, emotion, determination, memory, and imagination that takes place within the brain. Mind is often used to refer especially to the thought processes of reason.[30]

As with so many aspects of this inquiry, the debate of brain versus mind has been argued since the time of Aristotle and Plato and continues to this day.

Consciousness vs. Conscience

Consciousness and conscience are not the same and are indeed quite different. Consciousness (awareness) and conscience (morality) are two different concepts.[31] For centuries, philosophers and others have attempted, unsuccessfully, to define a single, acceptable definition of the human consciousness. For example, some standard definitions currently expressed in various dictionaries for the term *consciousness* include the following:

1. In Webster's Third New International Dictionary, they define consciousness as (in part): awareness or perception of an inward psychological or spiritual fact: intuitively perceived knowledge of something in one's inner self, inward awareness of an external object, state, or fact[32]
2. The state or activity that is characterized by sensation, emotion, *volition* (e.g., conscious choice), or thought, mind

---

[29] A. Satsaugi, "What is the difference between the mind and the brain?" https://www.researchgate.net/post/What_is_difference_between_mind_and_brain/4e737ebeffea752956000001/citation/download.

[30] Id.

[31] "Conscience," en.wikipedia.org/wiki/Conscience.

[32] "Consciousness," en.wikipedia.org/wiki/Consciousness.

in the broadest possible sense: something in nature that is distinguished from the physical[33]

3. The totality in psychology of sensations, perceptions, ideas, attitudes, and feelings of which an individual or a group is aware at any given time or within a particular time span[34]

The Cambridge Dictionary defines *consciousness* as the state of understanding and realizing something.[35] The Oxford Living Dictionary defines *consciousness* as the state of having perception of something and the fact of awareness by the mind of itself and the world.[36]

Stuart Sutherland presented a more skeptical definition of consciousness with his 1989 entry in the Macmillan Dictionary of Psychology wherein he stated:

Consciousness: The having of perceptions, thoughts, and feelings, awareness. The term is impossible to define except in terms that are unintelligible without a grasp of what consciousness means. Many fall into the trap of equating consciousness with self-consciousness—to be conscious it is only necessary to be aware of the external world.[37]

Conscience: can be described as producing feelings of remorse when a person does something that is out of character with their ethics, values, and morality. It is a cognitive process that brings forth emotions and feelings based upon the persons morals and values.[38]

---

[33] Id.
[34] Id.
[35] Id., Cambridge Dictionary.
[36] Id., The Oxford Living Dictionary.
[37] "Consciousness," en.wikipedia.org/wiki/Consciousness.
[38] "Conscience," en.wikipedia.org/wiki/Conscience.

Cognition: is defined as: the mental action or process of acquiring knowledge and understanding through experience, and the sense.[39]

Your consciousness is always aware, so it's impossible not to perceive something.[40]

Brain Implants

Brain implants, or neural implants, as they are often referred to, are devices or systems that establish a direct link between the brain and the electronic device. This system is typically used to stimulate a portion of the nervous system, thereby enabling the function of the brain to be modified, recorded, and/or translated for the manipulation of devices such as a computer cursor or a robotic arm.[41]

Some brain implants involve creating interfaces between neural systems and computer chips.[42] Interface technologies are divided into those that "read" the brain to record brain activity and decode its meaning and those that "write" to the brain to manipulate its process.[43]

Neurotechnology companies, like Neuralink, founded by Elon Musk in San Francisco, predict bidirectional coupling in which computers respond to people's brain activity and insert information into their neural activity in specific regions and affect their function.[44]

Frederic Gilbert, an ethicist who studies brain-computer interfaces (BCIs) at the University of Tasmania in Hobart, Australia, has stated that deep-brain stimulation (DBS), although very effective for certain treatments, also produces some serious side effects. Some patients

---

[39] "Cognition," en.wikipedia.org/wiki/Cognition.
[40] "Consciousness," en.wikipedia.org/wiki/Consciousness.
[41] A. Tyson, "Use of brain implants in humans," *Access Science.*
[42] "Brain Implants," en.wikipedia.org/wiki/Brain Implants.
[43] Id.
[44] L. Drew, "The ethics of brain – computer interfaces," https://www.nature.com/articles/d41586-019-02214-2.

have developed a distorted perception of themselves, offering the following comments: "You just wonder how much is you anymore. How much of it is my thought pattern? You feel kind of artificial."[45]

Gilbert believes that the DBS technology degrades people's ability to make decisions for themselves because someone other than the patient can potentially terminate treatment against the patient's wishes. It suggests that if a person thinks in a certain way only when an electrical current alters their brain activity, then those thoughts do not reflect an authentic self.[46]

The identified serious side effects, the potential vulnerability of such a neurological implanted device, and the unacceptable inherent risks associated with its use would appear to support the oversight scrutiny of neuroethicists. However, the inability of the subject neurological implantable device and its treatment would not have passed the scrutiny of the FDA to perform in a safe, effective, and reliable manner and thus would never have been approved by the Agency for use.

A neural device is implanted in the body and interacts with neurons.[47] Scientists speculate that in the future, neural implants could literally read and edit a person's thoughts.[48] Currently, these devices can treat disease, rehabilitate the body after injury, improve memory, and communicate with prosthetic limbs typically referred to as "mind-controlled prostheses."[49, 50]

These brain-implantable systems give amputees the unique ability to control the robotic movements of body extremities like the hands, arms, and legs by using their thoughts, again made possible

---

[45] Id.

[46] Id.

[47] E. Waltz, "How Do Neural Implants Work?" https://spectrum.ieee.org/the-human-os/biomedical/devices/what-is-neural-implant-neuromodulation-brain-implants-electroceuticals-neuralink-definitio.

[48] Id.

[49] E. Waltz, "How Do Neural Implants Work?" https://spectrum.ieee.org/the-human-os/biomedical/devices/what-is-neural-implant-neuromodulation-brain-implants-electroceuticals-neuralink-definitio.

[50] Id.

through neural implants.[51] In addition, this unique capability can enable the robotic arm, for example, to provide sensory feedback by stimulating nerves just above the amputation, giving the user a sense of what they are touching. Neural implants allow scientists to access the nervous system, which controls thinking, seeing, hearing, feeling, moving, and urinating. It also controls many involuntary processes such as organ function and the body's inflammatory, respiratory, cardiovascular, and immune systems.[52]

A typical surgical procedure for the implantation of a DBS system to treat some of the neurological deficiencies described previously would basically involve the following. During surgery, a hole is inserted into the patient's skull, and electrical leads are implanted directly into the brain's tissue. The leads are threaded out, and the skull is closed. These wires are threaded behind the ears, down the neck, and to the front chest area, where they are connected to a watch-sized device that emits a controlled amount of electricity. The entire unit, from wires to generator, is all buried just below the skin.[53] The patient can control the electrical dosage via a cell phone-sized remote control device, including the ability to turn the device on and off.[54]

According to the National Parkinson Foundation, these DBS surgical procedures can cost between $35,000 and $50,000. For a procedure involving both sides of the brain, the cost can range between $70,000 to $100,000.[55]

Selected brain stimulation can also establish new sensory pathways that can assist the blind or those who have lost their sense of touch.[56]

---

[51] Id.

[52] Id.

[53] M. Juang, "Advances in brain pacemaker reduces tremors, helps Parkinson's sufferers live a more normal life," https://www.cnbc.com/2017/10/05/brain-pacemaker-stops-tremors-helps-parkinsons-sufferers.html.

[54] Id.

[55] Id.

[56] A. Tyson, "Use of brain implants in humans," *Access Science*, https://doi.org/10.1036/1097-8542.YB160501.

According to neuroscientist Gene Civillico at the National Institute of Health (NIH), "Anything that the nervous system does could be helped or healed by an electrically active intervention—if we knew how to do it."[57]

The technology of these neural-implantable stimulation devices has advanced to a level more readily accepted in a science-fiction movie.

Scientists have demonstrated the ability of such devices to improve a patient's memory. **Yet more astonishing is the capability of these brain implants to operate computers and type sentences using only their thoughts and even determine a person's mood based on brain activity alone** (emphasis added).[58]

Such dramatic advancements with the improved capabilities of expanding the functional possibilities of the brain certainly stirs the imagination into yet new future areas that could increase a person's cognitive abilities, resulting in spectacular benefits for mankind. Future advancements may even permit the brain to initiate physical movements of a transplanted donor's body (corpse) from the transplanted brain thought its thought process. However, such speculative possibility is certainly beyond any near future expectation, if at all, especially when considering the enormous anatomical problems that must first be overcome.

Following are a few examples of brain-implanted electrical stimulation devices:

- **Neuroprostheses** are a series of devices that can substitute a motor, sensory, or cognitive modality (the employment of any therapeutic agent, limited usually to physical agents)[59]

---

[57] E. Waltz, "How Do Neural Implants Work? IEEE Spectrum," https://spectrum.ieee.org/the-human-os/biomedical/devices/what-is-neural-implant-neuromodulation-brain-implants-electroceuticals-neuralink-definitio.

[58] Id.

[59] "Modality," Medical Dictionary, 27th ed.

that might have been damaged as a result of an injury or a disease.[60]

- **Neurostimulators**, including deep brain stimulators, send electrical impulses to the brain to treat neurological and movement disorders, including Parkinson's disease, epilepsy, treatment-resistant depression, and other conditions such as urinary incontinence.[61] Electrodes are implanted into a specific part of the brain, connected via wires under the skin to a pacemaker-like stimulator in the chest. That pacemaker sends out electrical signals that stifle the part of the brain causing the tremors.[62]

- The **vagus nerve stimulator** (**VNS**) has been used to treat many inflammatory disorders, such as sepsis, lung injury, rheumatoid arthritis, and diabetes. It has also been used to control pain in fibromyalgia and migraines.[63] The vagus nerve is known as the wandering nerve because it has multiple branches that diverge from two thick stems rooted in the cerebellum (the part of the brain concerned in the coordination of movements)[64] and brain stem that wander to the lowest viscera (e.g., any large interior organ) of your abdomen, touching your heart and most major organs along the way. Vagus means *wandering* in Latin.[65]

- The **auditory brainstem implant** (**ABI**), an implanted electronic device, provides a sense of sound to a person who is

[60] "Artificial Organ," en.wikipedia.org/wiki/Artificial Organ.

[61] Id.

[62] A. Dance, "Scientists Want to Use Brain Implants to Tune the Mind," https://www.kavlifoundation.org/science-spotlights/scientists-want-use-brain-implants-tune-mind#.XxoEWJ5Kjcs.

[63] R. Johnson et al., "A review of vagus nerve stimulation as a therapeutic intervention," *Journal of Inflammation Research*, Doi:10.2147/JIR.S163248.

[64] "Cerebellum," Medical Dictionary, 27th ed.

[65] K. Tracey, "Vagus Nerve Stimulation Reduces Inflammation and the Systems of Arthritis," https://www.cesultra.com/blog/vagus-nerve-stimulation-reduces-inflammation-systms-arthritis-part-1/?gclid=EAlalQobChM19tWPOD r6lVQ77Ach.

profoundly deaf due to illness or injury damaging the cochlea (e.g., forms part of the inner ear)[66] or auditory nerve.[67]

- A **hippocampus prosthesis** is a cognitive-implanted device in the nervous system intended to improve or replace the function of damaged brain tissue.[68]

What Is the Function of a Neuron?

Neurons are responsible for carrying information throughout the human body. Using electrical and chemical signals, they help coordinate all of the necessary functions of life. In short, our nervous systems detect what is going on around us and inside of us; they decide how we should act, alter the state of internal organs (e.g., heart rate changes), and allow us to think about and remember what is going on. To do this, it relies on a sophisticated network, neurons.[69]

Consider the Following and Prepare to Be Astonished!

Most individuals have little or no appreciation for the enormous and unfathomable capability of the human brain to store information (e.g., memory capacity). For comparison, if your brain worked like a digital video recorder in a television, 2.5 petabytes would be enough to hold three million hours of TV shows. You would have to leave the TV running continuously for more than 300 years to use up all that storage.[70]

According to a 2010 article in *Scientific American*, the memory capacity of the human brain was reported to have the equivalent of

[66] "Cochlea," Medical Dictionary, 27th ed.
[67] "Auditory Brainstem Implant," en.wikipedia.org/wiki/Auditory Brainstem Implant.
[68] "Hippocampal prosthesis," en.wikipedia.org/wiki/Hippocampal prosthesis.
[69] T. Newan, "All you need to know about neurons," https://www.medicalnewstoday.com/articles/320289.
[70] P. Reber, "What is the Memory Capacity of the Human Brain," https://www.scientificamerican.com/article/what-is-the-memory-capacity.

2.5 petabytes of memory capacity. As a number, a petabyte means 1024 terabytes, or a million gigabytes, so the average adult human brain has the ability to store the equivalent of 2.5 million gigabytes of digital memory.[71]

For another astonishing example, consider the following. By comparison, the IRS's own massive data warehouse, which keeps track of 300-plus million Americans and many more million businesses, has the capacity of 150 terabytes of memory. Yet Yahoo's 2.0-petabyte computational center, which can process 24 billion events a day, **is a full 20 percent smaller than the capacity of a single human brain** (emphasis added).[72] It's difficult to fully comprehend.

Other compiled data report that the average human brain contains about 100 billion neurons that can be connected to up to 10,000 other neurons. There are as many as 1,000 trillion synaptic connections, equivalent to a computer with 1 trillion-bit-per-second processor. Modern home computers can perform at 4 gigahertz or higher, which is 4,000 million cycles per second.[73]

Therefore, the human brain has the ability to retain an almost-unlimited amount of information for as long as the brain continues to function. Scientists believed in the recent past that once we started to lose neurons, that would be it. We would be unable to create new brain cells.[74]

However, it turns out that this isn't true. Researcher Sandrine Thuret from King's College London in the United Kingdom has explained that the hippocampus is a crucial part in the adult brain in terms of generating new cells.[75]

---

[71] S. Smith, "What is the Memory Capacity of the Human Brain?" https://www. cnsnevada.com/what-is-the-memory-capacity-of-a-human-brain/#:-:text=As a number%2C a "petabyte,2.5 million gigabytes digital memory.

[72] Id.

[73] J. Hayward, "Fascinating Things About the Brain," https://www.activebeat.com/ your-health/9-fascinating-things-about-the-brain/?utm_medium=cpc&utm_ source=google_search_network&utmcampaign.

[74] M. Cohut, "Seven (or more) things you didn't know about your brain," *Medical News Today.*

[75] Id.

What Is Memory?

The memories we retain involve an overly complex process with an enormous amount of stored information and yet still avails additional storage capability without any apparent limitation, unlike most computers.

Understanding the essence of our memory remains somewhat a mystery to science. Nonetheless, our memories define who we are and, to a significant extent, our life. Memory involves the process of acquiring, storing, retaining, and later retrieving information.[76] Human memory is the ability to preserve and recover information we have learned or experienced.[77]

Memory is stored information, much of which we are not aware of except for times when we must recover certain information we have previously stored (e.g., while studying for an exam) and subsequently drawing upon certain information during the time of the exam. Thus, most of our stored memory is usually outside our awareness. The retrieval process recovers stored information from our memories and converts it into conscious awareness.[78]

We can build upon our stored long-term memory. For example, when we decide to take up a sport, like skiing or tennis, our initial attempts demonstrate our lack of proficiency and poor skill level. However, with repeated attempts, our ability to master the sport increases because our long-term memory has been strengthened to the extent that we naturally improve without thinking about it.

Our brain has learned how to effectively increase and coordinate the various muscles required to function at a greater skill level. This is often referred to as muscle memory. We also witness the effectiveness of reinforced and repetitive processes in sports teams. Not discounting the natural skill level of team members, why do some teams and individual members play better than others do? A

---

[76] K. Cherry. "What Is Memory? Cognitive Psychology," https://www.verywellmind.com/what-is-memory-2795006.

[77] Id.

[78] Id.

good coach will be more effective in training their individual team members and the team as a whole, with a more effective method of improving their long-term memory and recall response to an anticipated situation on the field.

A highly qualified sports player, especially at the rookie level, will produce on the field at different levels of ability based upon how effective their physical and especially their mental training will be. Depending upon the skill, motivation, and experience of their coaches and their ability to effectively interact with their team members, the long-term memory learning experience will translate to different levels of proficiency on the field.

For example, a rookie has been drafted from a university after demonstrating an unusually high level of athleticism and proficiency during their college years of playing. The rookie is now part of a professional team and is full of enthusiasm and eagerness to get on the field to support the team and demonstrate their ability to perform at the professional level.

Now, the rookie arrives at their first day at training camp at a particular skill level, both physically and mentally. Their eventual success will be determined in large part by the ability of their coach to increase (or potentially decrease) their success on the playing field.

An outstanding example of this was demonstrated during the 1980 Winter Olympic Games at Lake Placid when the recently-amalgamated U.S. hockey team was formed with players from various parts of the country who came together for the first time to train. These were young American boys destined to face the heavily-favored Soviet hockey team, considered to be more of a professional team and believed to easily win the gold medal in hockey.

When Herb Brooks initially received his team members for training at Lake Placid, he realized they were a rather dysfunctional team lacking any cohesive structure. The film *Miracle on Ice* effectively depicts what could be accomplished by a dynamic and determined coach even when the odds clearly depict the task to be accomplished as near impossible.

Herb Brooks was incredibly effective in his dynamic ability to recognize the individual mental processes of his team members that lacked focus and even team spirit. However, he recognized that his team did have the potential to accomplish great things if he could properly train them to accept the apparent impossible challenges they would eventually face against tough opponents, especially the Russians.

More concerning to Herb than the enormous physical challenges of training were the mental and emotional challenges to overcome within his team. Eventually, as the movie depicted, Herb was able to instill within each player and ultimately the team by repetitive training and a mental focus so strong that their effectiveness on the ice became an almost automatic memory response at peak performance.

As a sidebar, I attended the 1980 Winter Olympic games and actually had tickets for both my wife and I to attend the hockey game between the U.S. team and the Russians. However, since there was so much negative press about the inability of the American high school hockey team facing the Russians and the ultimate embarrassment of a dramatic loss to the Soviets, we decided to exchange the hockey tickets for a ski event. To this day, I cannot believe I did that, an ultimate example of regrettable hindsight!

I said all of this to simply illustrate that the human brain has the innate and incredible ability to be receptive to coherent cognitive input and storage. To a large extent, the ultimate quality and potential to effectively coordinate one's life on a daily basis will be dependent upon the source of the stored memory, the level of cognitive retention of stored information, and the ability to effectively retrieve appropriate information at the time needed.

We ultimately become who we are by the exposure we have to other individuals and circumstances starting at the earliest time of life as infants when we absorb our environment and the input we receive from those who care for us, especially our mothers and usually to a lesser extent our fathers.

Unfortunately, our memory stores information received from individuals with whom we had no ability to censor, or select, as most qualified and appropriate to provide the most advantageous information for storage and retrieval. This is not the world we live in—never has been and most likely never will be.

Throughout the entirety of our lives, especially during our younger years, we have functioned like memory-recording devices subjected to a continued, nonstop, and often-unwanted input of information being installed in our memory. From family members, teachers, friends, employers, and even TV—the good, the bad, and the ugly—we take it in and store these unfiltered experiences in our memory.

Thus, the input of information that floods from our life experiences is not provided with a screening mechanism that would sift out undesirable information and events. The younger we are, the more readily we absorb and store all incoming information that eventually produces the uniqueness of who we turn out to be. Starting during our earliest years, effectively involving the imprinting years, all incoming information is readily processed without question or concern, no matter how polluted the information is going into storage.

However, as we grow older and experience the trials and tribulations of life, including the positive prior experiences, we become more discerning and hesitant to readily accept all incoming information at face value. We become more inquisitive and judgmental when processing new information, and at the same time, we begin to formulate our personal opinions on the subject based upon our prior exposure to the topic and therefore become more predisposed to a natural inclination, belief, attitude, disposition, temperament, or preference.

When we are born, our cognitive potential (the essence of who we will become) is like fresh clay placed upon a potter's wheel, awaiting its destiny to be determined by those who will place their hands upon the new clay and start the manipulation process of constructing our evolving psyche. What we are all ultimately left with is a belief system, opinions, attitudes, temperament, fears, aspirations, inhibitions, and our own individual spectrum of uniquely stored behavior patterns in our memory that, for better or worse, we will recall in response to any situation that arises as we attempt to navigate our way through daily life.

It has been our cognitive exposure and retention of the enormous amount of varied input into our psyche that has ultimately caused us to react in the manner we do to any given situation. For example, and to the extreme, why has there been such deeply entrenched and varied emotional outbursts during the political interactions between the Democratic and Republican parties during 2020 and 2021 period and especially involving their various support groups? What specific imprinting factors occurred, especially during our formative years, that became so significant to cause such strong and unyielding opinions?

Think back to a time when you can identify certain individuals whom you believe influenced your life the most and in some manner formulated your attitude and perspective about responding to life's varied circumstances. You may be able to identify several individuals whom you believe had the greatest influence in the manner that you address conflict issues or that contributed to you being more of an introvert or extrovert or especially sensitive to certain issues or even your basic likes and dislikes.

In the vast majority of cases, each of us was born into life and exposed by happenstance from the very beginning of our existence to parents and family members not of our own choosing. The spectrum of our vulnerability to the quality of our being reared will avail a divergence from very loving and caring parents to the other extreme end of the spectrum. Most of us will reside somewhere in between.

The point being made here is that, for the most part, we were not involved with the formation of our own attitudes and perspectives. Eventually we may become aware of certain feelings we recognize within our being that may portray an unwanted character flaw or perspective on certain life issues. Many individuals remain so troubled by such concerns that they seek the help of a psychiatrist in hopes of reconciling their mental concern and problematic memories.

In 1968, Richard Atkinson and Richard Shiffrin described three individual stages of memory: sensory memory, short-term memory, and long-term memory.[79] Each of these can be distinguished based on storage capacity and duration.[80]

Sensory memory is the earliest stage of memory. During this stage, sensory information from the environment is stored for a very brief period, generally for no longer than half-second for visual information and three or four seconds for auditory information.[81]

Short-term memory, also known as active memory, is the information we are currently aware of or thinking about. Most of the information stored in active memory will be kept for approximately twenty to thirty seconds.[82] This has to do with your brain's capacity for holding small amounts of information in the active mind. The brain keeps this information in an available state for easy access, but only does so for about a minute and a half. Most people hold memory for numbers for about seven seconds and memory for letters about nine seconds.[83]

Short-term memory is profoundly affected by time duration or interruption on the short-term focus. In other words, if you are trying to remember a phone number a friend gave you a moment ago and you are interrupted or distracted while walking to your car, you will most likely forget the number. The most significant detriments to maintaining short-term memory, or thoughts, is lack of focus and distractions. Our brains have not evolved for short-term memory to function beyond a brief moment of recall in order to accomplish an immediate task.

Long-term memory refers to the continuing storage of information. This information is largely outside of our awareness but can be called into working memory to be used when needed.[84] I

---

[79] Id.

[80] K. Cherry, "Short-Term Memory Duration and Capacity," https://www.verywellmind.com/ what-is-short-term-memory-2795348.

[81] K. Cherry, "What Is Memory-Sensory Memory," https://www.verywellmind.com/what-is-memory-2795066.

[82] Id.

[83] Dent Neurologic Institute, "22 Facts About the Brain."

[84] K. Cherry, "What Is Memory: Long-Term Memory," https://www.verywellmind.com/what-is-memory-2795066.

am amazed at the ability I have to retrieve long-term memory events and with such detail and clarity. For example, I can recall a moment when I was two years old living in a row house in Philadelphia and playing in the small backyard. I can remember the flowers and even their bright colors.

I can also identify a time when I was about six when we had an icebox for a refrigerator. Mom would place a sign in the window to inform the ice man the size of ice that she wanted for the icebox (e.g., fifteen- or twenty-five-cent piece). Along with the other kids in the neighborhood, I would grab small pieces of ice from the back of the ice truck. Many other childhood memories are quickly retrievable as well. All of us had the experience of retrieving a memory initiated from one of our five basic senses, for example, the sight of a photo, the sound of a song, the smell of a fragrance, the taste of a meal, or the touch of certain material, and so on.

Long-term memory tends to remain stable and is easily retrievable and accurate. Also, memories stored during a highly emotional experience, either good or bad, will be easier to retrieve than others. Emotion plays an important role in storing memory. The stronger the feelings experienced and stored in the memory, the easier it will be to recall this information later.

Take a moment to travel back in time to the earliest moment you can remember. Notice how young you were and how vivid your recall is of that moment in time. It may reflect a special occasion or maybe a detail that did not seem particularly significant at the time, yet it has been stored as a long-term memory.

Have you ever had a conversation with an old classmate or family member about prior experiences at an earlier time in your lives? Your back-and-forth discussion would have brought out memories that were not previously part of your conscious thoughts. The storage capacity of your long term-memory and your ability to retrieve the smallest detail from memory involves an astonishing capability of the brain.

Also, the next time you are writing something, notice how the words you are writing seems to form and flow effortlessly. You are not concentrating on the formation of each letter or word and perhaps not focusing on the subject matter much either, and yet the words appear almost automatically. This is a form of prior programmed memory learning, similar to talking or walking, which are retrieved from long-term memory, and prior experiences learned especially during the early years of your life.

Consider the ability of the brain to transfer your message intent from the brain to your fingertips and to generate the dexterity and movement necessary for you to write your message with little forethought. It is truly an amazing process that we all take for granted.

There is a dramatic difference in duration of time between short- and long-term memory. Short-term memory has the limited ability to store memory for a very short period and a minimal amount of information. **Conversely, long-term memory is thought to have no limits and a storage capacity considered unlimited. According to some studies, the upper bound on the size of visual and acoustic long-term memory has not been reached** (emphasis added).[85]

Memory Loss

As we age, we experience more apparent memory problems, especially involving short-term memory. These can range from minor concerns like forgetting where we placed our keys to far more significant concerns involving Alzheimer's and dementia, which affect the quality of life and the ability to function effectively.

Irreversible long-term memory deficits include Alzheimer's disease and dementia. Alzheimer's disease causes memory loss and difficulty in comprehension, reasoning, and judgment. Dementia's first system is short-term memory loss, which is then followed by long-term memory loss.[86]

The terms *Alzheimer's* and *dementia* have been around for more than a century, which means people have likely been mixing them

---

[85] "The Human Memory," htpps://human-memory.net/long-term-memory.
[86] Id.

up for that long too. But knowing the difference is important. One is broader than the other. If placed side by side, Alzheimer's would fit inside dementia, accounting for an estimated 60 to 80 percent of cases.[87]

Dementia is a decline in mental function that is usually irreversible. It's a syndrome, not a disease, notes Ron Petersen, director of the Mayo Clinic Alzheimer's Disease Research Center at the Mayo Clinic Study of Aging in Rochester, Minnesota. To be called dementia, the disorder must be severe enough to interfere with your daily life, says psychiatrist Constantine George Lyketsos, director of the John Hopkins Memory and Alzheimer's Treatment Center in Baltimore. The earliest stage of dementia, known as mild cognitive impairment, is considered "forgetfulness beyond what is expected from aging," according to Director Ron Petersen at the Mayo Clinic.[88]

Alzheimer's is a specific brain disease that progressively and irreversibly destroys memory and thinking skills. Age is the biggest risk factor for the disease. Eventually, Alzheimer's disease removes the ability to carry out even the simplest tasks.[89]

Causes of Memory Loss

Some of the more common causes of memory loss include medications. Both prescription and over-the-counter drugs, including antidepressants, antihistamines, antianxiety drugs, muscle relaxants, tranquilizers, sleeping pills, and after-surgery pain medications, can cause memory loss.[90] Other causes include alcohol, tobacco, sleep deprivation, depression and stress, nutritional deficiency, head injury, and stroke.

Normal aging is associated with a decline in various memory abilities in many cognitive tasks; the phenomenon is known as age-related memory impairment (AMI) or age-associated memory

---

[87] K. Fifield, "Dementia vs. Alzheimer's: Which Is It?" https://www.aarp.org/health/dementia/info-2018/difference-between-dementia-alzheimers.
[88] Id.
[89] Id.
[90] C. Melinosky, "Memory Loss," https://www.webmdcom/brain/memory-loss#1-2.

EDWARD W. REESE, PH.D.

impairment (AAMI). The deficits may be related to impairments observed in the ability to refresh recently processed information.[91]

Source information is one type of episodic memory that suffers with old age; this kind of knowledge includes where and when the person learned the information. Knowing the source and context of information can be extremely important in daily decision-making, so this is one way in which memory decline can affect the lives of the elderly.

Many studies have tested psychologist theories throughout the years, and they have found solid evidence that supports older adults having a harder time recalling contextual information while the more familiar or automatic information typically stays well-preserved throughout the aging process. Also, there is an increase in irrelevant information as one ages, which can lead to an elderly person believing false information since they are often in a state of confusion.[92]

To the extent that someone experiences memory loss, from a mild cognitive impairment to complete loss of any cognitive function, will also equate to the extent of their awareness.

Forget Something?

Forgetting is an everyday normal occurrence for most people. Have you ever walked into a room, stopped, and tried to remember what you were looking for or forget the name of a prior acquaintance who you are about to meet?

Preoccupied with Other Thoughts?

Has it come to your attention lately that you are becoming more forgetful more often? Are you wondering if maybe you are experiencing the onset of dementia or Alzheimer's disease? In most cases, you have little to worry about.

---

[91] "Memory and Aging," enwikipedia.org/wiki/MemoryandAging.
[92] Id.

Most people are usually preoccupied with some matter or another. For example, I have noticed that when I am heavily involved in a project, my thinking will often proceed my physical focus and attention. I will often place an item I am working with on the table when I have finished with it and moved on with my project, only to wonder where I put the object when I need it again. My focus on the object I placed down had a lower priority at the time than did my project, which moved on with no further attention for the abandoned item and the completion of the prior task.

This aspect of managing my projects had become so frustrating and disorienting to my focus and train of thought that I finally decided to address the distraction by taking a moment whenever I was finished with an item during my project to physically take note of where I was placing the item, sometimes pointing to it to solidify the moment of focus.

You may notice that you have been particularly preoccupied when you are troubled about a serious problem relating to a relationship, health, work, finances, or any matter is causing you to overly dwell on the problem. I have also experienced negative consequences associated with prolonged mental processing of a problem or dilemma over and over again, especially when a solution or resolution to the problem was not at hand. This can be called "stubborn thinking" where the tendency is to refuse giving up on an inability to reconcile the issue and move on.

As a researcher, I want to identify a solution to a particular problem that usually requires a resolution before I can move forward and build upon previously established findings; however, in the real world, this is not how we move forward in our understanding of scientific discovery and advancement. Many times, it is necessary to leave a certain problem unresolved and move forward to other areas of study, which can provide new insights that enable me to go back to the unresolved problem and reach a satisfactory conclusion.

Eventually I arrived at a solution that works for me, although it took considerable effort to reject or resist the old nature to stubbornly, repeatedly, and persistently work on resolving the problem even when it was apparent that no reasonable or acceptable solution was possible or forthcoming at the time. I ultimately determined that while I must be responsible for investing as much of me into any research project or investigation as I deemed appropriate, at some point thereafter, it was necessary for me to move on to new projects and challenges. At that point, I end the frustration by thinking, *Well, that's all of me that you can have, at least for now.*

Of course, it does not require serious scientific research topics to preoccupy your thoughts to the extent that you lose focus on your surroundings, task, or objectives. You could forget what you wanted to get from the pantry because you're thinking about preparing the remainder of the meal.

This process should work involving any problematic circumstance, especially as it pertains to those matters you deem serious and hinder your life in one manner or another. For example, if you are having a relationship problem with a friend, family member, or work employee that never seems to get resolved, eventually you may get to a point where you determine that you are willing to initiate some additional activities and efforts and thus hope for some acceptable level of resolution. However, beyond that point where you believe you have been responsible for investing the appropriate effort to resolve the dilemma, you should recognize that you must then move forward with your life and leave the issue behind. "That's all of me that you can have!"

It's time to reinvest the unresolved mental focus and frustration into matters more beneficial to your life. Easier said than done, I know, but to bury yourself in attempts to resolve a difficulty, especially involving personal relationship issues that constantly throw up barriers of discontent, will keep you in a dysfunctional and ineffective realm of unhappiness, depression, and frustration. This is a defeated existence of your awareness and well-being that you should recognize must come to an end.

I realize this approach may seem harsh and mechanical; nonetheless, its intent is to result in freedom for your mind in order to grow and become more productive. In a way, it's like spending money to constantly repair the car you loved and owned for many years, even when the mechanic informs you that the vehicle is far past its useful existence. There comes a point when you must finally decide to let it go. I know it's a big difference between letting the car go and a friendship, but you get the point.

If you are having repeated daily experiences with forgetfulness and you are aware of being preoccupied at the time, develop an appropriate response to preclude being preoccupied, such as my previous example or whatever process works for you. Make a reasonable effort to take charge of the problem and eliminate or, at a minimum, reduce its negative impact on your life.

Another lapse of memory, or more appropriately stated, lapse of focus, I experienced almost every week involved my forgetting to take out the trash on Sunday night for a Monday morning pickup. I found that a simple self-imposed reminder was very effective, not just as a reminder to take out the trash but other activities that required a prompt. For example, while watching TV at the end of the day, I would crumble a piece of paper and place it on the carpet before my chair. When I got up to go to bed, the ball of crumbled paper reminded me to take out the trash.

We all have experienced processing problems that preoccupy our thoughts when we place our head upon the pillow at bedtime. These reflect unresolved or pending concerns that we deem serious enough to hinder our sleep and peace of mind. Often these more problematic preoccupations will carry on day after day and night after night because it is assumed to be overly difficult to implement any appropriate resolution or corrective measure or simply because there is fear of the unknown or apprehension and dread that a wrong response will result in greater issues to be resolved. In other words, fear to act and the unknown are the great inhibitors to resolving the many serious problems of life. Also, these troubling thoughts that keep you awake at night or cause you to lose focus during the day are especially problematic when the cause of such concerns does not appear to provide a remedy to effectively address the concern.

For example, your company has hired a new manager to replace your current one. Your first impression of the new manager is not favorable, and there are rumors that they may want to replace some staff members with their own people. You now feel vulnerable and find yourself continually preoccupied, day and night, with the fear you may lose your job. This illustrates a fearful preoccupation of mental awareness and focus that most individuals have experienced at some points of their life. During the times when one is living through such fearful concerns that could dramatically affect their well-being and their family, the focus of the involved person can be so dramatic that until the concern is resolved, one way or another, it will continue to inhibit their ability to move forward in a fully productive manner.

Elizabeth Loftus is a memory researcher who has identified four major reasons why people forget: retrieval failure, interference, failure to store, and motivated forgetting.[93]

Retrieval Failure

One possible cause is identified as decay theory, which explains that memory begins to fade and disappear over time. If the information is not retrieved and rehearsed, it will eventually be lost.[94] Nonetheless, research has determined that even memories that have not been rehearsed or remembered are remarkably stable in long-term memory.[95] For example, my ninety-six-year-old mother could recite in very graphic detail her childhood experiences in Philadelphia, although her short-term memory was problematic.

Interference

This theory suggests that some memories compete and interfere with other memories. When information is similar to other information that was previously stored in memory, interference is

---

[93] K. Cherry, "4 Explanations for Why We Forget," https://www.verywellmind.com/explanations-for-forgetting-2795054.

[94] Id.

[95] Id.

CAN YOU LIVE FOREVER?

more likely to occur.[96] Another problem that causes forgetfulness is lack of focus or a wandering mind. A common occurrence involving both distractions usually becomes apparent during your mental idle time when you are driving to and from work over a repetitive route. For example, your stored memory may drift away from where you intend to go to thoughts of how you intend to spend the weekend or problems that need to be addressed while subconsciously you continue to your destination, to the extreme you may find yourself driving to a common destination when suddenly you cannot recall the directions because you were so locked into your wandering thoughts. Only when you are required to turn right or left are you snapped back into the immediate need to recover the stored memory that will remind you of where you intended to go and to make the appropriate turn.

Or perhaps you were studying for an exam the next day and had trouble preparing because you were unable to focus upon the material anticipated to be in the exam. In other words, you failed to effectively lock in sufficient information in your memory storage for retrieval to answer the anticipated question or problem.

Do not be overly concerned because such forgetfulness is a common occurrence with almost everyone, at any age, although more prevalent as we age. Some stored memories are effectively secured in your memory because such remembrances involve a special event that is easy to retrieve, for example, getting married, having a first child, or graduating, special days in your life when you experienced great joy or excitement. These events are typically pulled from your long-term memory storage files.

Failure to Store

It is not the amount of time you invest in preparing for the exam, but rather the quality of your focused attention to the subject matter you study. You could literally spend hours reviewing the prerequisite

---

[96] Id.

material and not absorb most or perhaps any of the study subject, depending on the strength of your focus or lack of sufficient focus.

In essence, what you have done is subconsciously place a higher priority, or greater emphasis, upon an unresolved problem or a circumstance, causing you to drift away from your study material. Of course, being physically or mentally tired would also diminish your ability to effectively store sufficient information required for the exam.

Some individuals can study with the TV on with other people milling around the room. Others require a quiet room with no distractions in order to maintain their focus and to maximize the retention of the studied material.

To effectively store the material being studied often requires repeated review of the same material, especially if one is tired or has difficulty focusing upon the text. Some individuals can store in their memory the required details and information more effectively than others can. The more effective the ability to concentrate and focus, the more effective the information is stored. If the mind drifts to other issues or concerns, the quality of storing and retrieving information will be diminished, perhaps dramatically.

Motivated Forgetting

When an individual has experienced a traumatic event in their past, they may strongly desire to erase or at least diminish the remembrance of the painful memory. The two basic forms of motivated forgetting are suppression, a conscious form of forgetting, and repression, an unconscious form of forgetting.[97]

Attempting to recall information or a situation that has occurred can be very difficult since different pieces of information of any particular event are stored in different areas of the brain. During recall of an event, the various pieces of information are placed back together, and any missing information is filled up by our brain

---

[97] Id.

unconsciously, which can account for us receiving and believing false information.[98]

Memory lapses can be both aggravating and frustrating, but they are due to the overwhelming number of details and information being taken in by the brain. Issues in memory can also be linked to several common physical and psychological causes, such as anxiety, dehydration, depression, infections, medication side effects, poor nutrition, vitamin B_{12} deficiency, psychological stress, substance abuse, chronic alcoholism, thyroid imbalances, and blood clots in the brain.[99]

I have one final reference to our preoccupied mind and distractions. Metaphorically speaking, imagine that at your birth, you were issued a backpack into which you were to deposit your life experiences as you matured. As the years went by, you effectively placed all your relevant experiences into the backpack, including both the good and the bad, without filtering either. Over time, you noticed the backpack was becoming heavier and heavier to the point where it was now becoming a significant burden. To reduce the painful load, you eventually decide to remove the backpack, open it, and determine if there are some items you could remove to reduce the burden upon your continued journey through life.

To your surprise, you notice a significant amount of tangible, bad experiences and traumatic events from your past life taking up a lot of space and contributing to your increased burden as you attempt to maneuver your way through life. You thus decide to remove and discard as many of these negative factors as possible that have previously hindered and inhibited your happiness and your ability to live a more productive life. While you were unable to remove all of the nonproductive and painful burdens from your backpack, you were successful in removing enough to continue your walk through life with a greater focus on reaching important goals in your life that were heretofore in doubt and with greater clarity of thought.

---

[98] "Memory and Aging," en.wikipedia.org/wiki/memory and aging.
[99] Id.

I said all that to simply illustrate a significant reality of life for the vast majority of individuals who have not removed their backpacks in order to review the problematic events during their past life's history, but rather decided to continue their life's journey while they begrudgingly ignored aspects of their past that hold them back and continue to cause unhappiness, depression, lack of motivation, and a sense of hopelessness.

Moreover, many of these individuals will continue to deposit additional burdens into their backpacks through the remainder of their life, not realizing that many of their past negative long-term stored memories could be reconciled to at least reduce the heavy load. Easier said than done, I realize, but for most of us, there comes a point in our life when it's time to take the backpack off and see what is inside.

The Learning Process

In 1949, psychologist Donald Hebb adapted Pavlov's associative learning rule to explain how brain cells might acquire knowledge. Hebb proposed that when two neurons fire together, sending off impulses simultaneously, the connections between them, the synapse, grow stronger. When this happens, learning has taken place.[100]

During the last two decades, neuroscientists have dramatically expanded their understanding of how the learning process occurs. Neuroscientists have long believed that learning and memory formation is made by the strengthening and weakening of connections among brain cells. Recently, researchers at the University of California Irvine's Center for the Neurobiology of Learning and Memory proved it. In experiments with mice, they were able to isolate and observe the actions of the brain while learning a new task.[101]

---

[100] R. Fields, "The Brain Learns in Unexpected Ways," https://www. scientificamerican.com/article/the-brain-learns-in-unexpected-ways/#:-text= In 1949 psychologist Donald Hebb, happens%2C learning ha.
[101] D. Ford, "How the Brain Learns," *Training Industry*.

When learning new things, frequency and recency strengthen memory and recall. The more we practice and rehearse something new and the more recently we have practiced, the easier it is for our brain to transmit these experiences efficiently and store them for ready access later.[102]

We all have experienced the learning process throughout our life, whether at school, work, military, or sports, involving focused study or training or through individuals and group interactions pertaining to less tangible experiences. Often it was necessary to repeatedly study the same material over multiple times until you were comfortable that your retention (memory storage) of the subject matter was adequate, at least to a reasonable extent. Like preparing for an Olympic event or the military or training repeatedly for acceptance within the Special Forces or the SEALS, such strong focus will often produce what is referred to as "muscle memory." In other words, the constant and continued repetition of the same training emphasis will enable a somewhat automatic and easier memory response to repeat the subject activity with minimal forethought in recalling from memory the appropriate response.

Perhaps the ultimate example of how effective muscle memory can respond to a particular situation has been experienced by military personnel involved in combat. Even when the thinking process is emotionally overwhelmed with fear and confusion, the memory of their prior vigorous training, firmly embedded in their memory, will respond in an appropriate manner to the situation with little or no focused decision-making as to what they should do.

Of course, much less emphasis with study or training will also enable our memory retrieval capability to accomplish an appropriate response, although lacking the extent of muscle memory referred to above. For example, there are repetitive activities that we perform routinely every day that have become so deep-seated within our memory that no concentrated emphasis on thinking about performing the task is necessary, like driving to work or school.

---

[102] Id.

To Learn Without Study or Training

Neuroscientists have researched the learning process at the molecular level, resulting in an ever-expanding understanding of how learning occurs and the molecular details of how synapses change during learning have been described in detail.[103] Neuroscientists, medical scientists, and other related brain specialists have continued to advance their understanding of how the brain is able to function in the manner it does. Their insights and knowledge of the brain's activity and capabilities are increasing and accelerating as they probe ever deeper to discover a more comprehensive understanding of its actual and potential capabilities.

As I extrapolate the historic advancements by scientists who have dedicated their expertise to unraveling the mysteries of the brain and the mind and look to the future of potential achievements, a dramatic and astonishing possibility emerges.

Prediction

I perceive and speculate that one day in the future, research scientists will ultimately understand how to artificially replicate the natural learning process involving the connection with brain cells and the firing of neurons and the synapse connections between them that produce learning to the extent that the time-consuming, arduous task and tedious repetition of study and even training will no longer be required or at least greatly minimized.

The transfer or injection of new data and information into the brain in an artificial manner is basically the opposite of the speculative futuristic process of uploading the existing contents of the brain into computers. (See section on "Human Consciousness Uploading/Downloading to a Computer or Artificial Brain.") Thus, potentially sometime in the future, scientists will have the ability to send and receive information to and even from the brain, utilizing this process.

---

[103] R. Fields, "The Brain Learns in Unexpected Ways."

Current neurological science and research speculation indicates it will eventually be possible for future students to select a subject they desire to pursue for a career and have the required prerequisite academic material artificially transferred into their brains. This would also include other non-academic individuals to also receive information to perform tasks that again would require significant study or training time to qualify for their selected field of expertise. For example, a student wanting a career in physics or accounting would be able to have the required learning experience delivered to their brain almost instantly or within a relatively short period of time. A military pilot could learn how to fly a helicopter through the same brain induction manner.

I anticipate there would be substantial prerequisites for such individuals prior to receiving the transfer of their desired academic pursuit or other areas of expertise. Also, governing bodies would have appropriate regulations in place to optimize safety and efficacy concerns. Moreover, I believe there would be imposed limitations on certain subjects that would be available to students or others in order to tailor the appropriate disbursement into society, the military, government, and so forth as such needs are determined.

I realize this sounds like some very futuristic science-fiction movie, as did many of the technology products available to us today did in the past. This future capability of near-instant learning will not occur overnight. It will undoubtedly require a lengthy period of scientific development, clinical study, and regulatory scrutiny by some controlling agency like our current FDA or some other governmental agency.

This is not to suggest that our schools of higher learning and other teaching institutions would cease to exist. They would not. I anticipate that the traditional ways of learning at colleges, universities, and so forth would continue their programs since those who would be recipients of brain-induced learning would involve a small number of individuals and not cause any significant reduction in the school's population.

I would not expect the availability of such instant learning as appropriate or available to everyone, but rather to a select few who could first afford the high cost of such a procedure and to those who could pass the prerequisite requirements involving their existing health (both physical and neurological) and the various agency regulatory requirements and so forth that would be imposed.

Moreover, I would not expect any such brain transfer of knowledge to be legally available to those in the traditional grades first through twelfth (or younger than a predetermined age) because these are the years when personal traits are learned and the intrinsic characteristics and values of the person are formed that make us individually unique. To do otherwise would then venture outside the intent of providing pure knowledge to appropriate candidates and into the realm of mind control and alterations that portend trouble in many areas of life. As with many advances in technology, there exists the real potential for illegal, destructive, and hazardous use.

Why Do I Not Like Them?

Often when one initially meets someone for the first time, they form a negative impression for reasons often not understood. Or there may be some aspect of the individual's appearance, verbal tone, or physical demeanor that elicits a less-than-favorable impression. Usually, these first impressions are quickly formed, perhaps even before you initiate any conversation with the individual.

Your discernment may be based upon your memory of a past traumatic or unpleasant experience recalled by some aspect of your past life experience or observation when meeting this individual. Or the factors that generate your unfavorable impression may be buried in your subconscious without bringing forth any obvious past recollection of a prior cause for your negative impression.

Of course, the opposite impression of warmth, appreciation, and acceptance can also be experienced when we first meet an individual we feel drawn to. Most of us have had similar experiences and accept our initial impressions without processing why do I feel this way about this stranger whom I just meet.

The observations initially formed when meeting someone for the first time are based upon the multitude of our various life experiences and are subconsciously evaluated and summarized based on the idiosyncrasies of who we are at any given point in our evolving life cycle. Some memories are based upon a lasting impression, both positive and negative, or more often stored from memorable experiences encountered through our daily lives.

The amalgamation of all these uniquely stored inputs into our memory are more fluid in our younger years when we are more accepting of issues that have not previously been adequately experienced in life. During the learning and inquisitive years of youth, the experiences involving a broad spectrum of living life will form many lasting memories more entrenched within our psyche.

It is only when one arrives at a point in life, when they begin to challenge some of the teachings, learnings, and life experiences that continue to provide data and information into their memory, that stored memory is more selective and refined rather than just accepted without challenge. Thus, our individually formulated and stored memory produces the unique person we have come to be, good or bad, like it or not. Consider for a moment the significance of that reality.

Humanity has not been provided with the opportunity of selective input into our evolving memory that would combine to form the unique characteristics of who we would desire to be. For the most part, we have had very little to say about how we would desire to formulate and hold true to our own opinions, beliefs, feelings, sensitivities, concerns, values, perspectives, and so forth. This learning process begins to form at a very early age when behavior patterns are established through daily contact with parents, teachers, friends, and other influential associations. These early learning experiences typically establish a more permanent perspective regarding how we perceive and respond to the daily experiences of living life.

So as we wonder through life, at any given age, our individual perspective about almost any issue, for the most part, will elicit either a thinking response and/or a physical response dependent upon how we subconsciously interpret and analyze the situation based upon how our memories were formulated.

It is not my intent to make this issue more complicated than it really is, so in other words, when considering the question, "Why do I not like them?" or "Why do I hold so fervently to certain opinions?" our internal mind computer will process our amalgamated stored memories in such a manner to determine, almost instantaneously, our most appropriate response to any given circumstance. This is not to suggest that the chosen response is right or wrong or appropriate or inappropriate. That is not the issue. It is the uniqueness of how life's experiences have combined and coalesced within an individual in such a manner that produces the given response as appropriate to a particular circumstance and the individual involved.

For example, recently in a suburb of Minneapolis, a driver was shot and killed as a result of road rage simply because he pulled in front of the assailant's vehicle, causing him to slow down. This apparently enraged the assailant. Try to imagine what circumstances conspired within the life of the assailant that resulted in his action to shoot and kill an innocent driver because he was momentarily inconvenienced.

For broader example, during the 2020 presidential election, the enthusiasm and demonstrations by both parties were so overtly aggressive that each side resorted to lawless action to further support their agenda. Such was the deeply entrenched and compassionate feeling of both parties and their supporters.

What has caused some people to become a Democrat or a Republican? Why do some love a Chevy versus a Ford? Why do some support gun legislation and others oppose it? Why are some Catholics and others Protestants? And the comparisons go on and on. Many individuals would have difficulty describing why they retain certain opinions or perspectives one way or another or why have they become the person they are. Why have some persons become criminals while others become ministers?

The answer, in most cases, is that we have inadvertently become who we are due to the accidental and unintended exposure of our being, our awareness, especially during the early years, to an environment and circumstances that were initially not of our own making.

Clarifying Common Related Terms (Definitions)

In addition to the discussion pertaining to the brain, mind, and memory, there are many other common references used when referring to the function of the brain. Therefore, let's briefly clarify the appropriate definition and function of these terms often used inappropriately or inaccurately. These common everyday terms and others include the following:

- Awareness is the state of being conscious of something. More specifically, it is the ability to personally know and perceive, to feel, or to be cognizant of events. The concept is often synonymous and also understood as being consciousness itself.[104] Awareness is also the knowledge that something exists or understanding of a situation or subject at the present time based on information or experience.[105] There are two normal states of awareness: consciousness and unconsciousness.[106] Self-awareness is the experience of one's own personality or individuality. It is not to be confused with consciousness. While consciousness is being aware of one's environment, body, and lifestyle, self-awareness is the recognition of that awareness. Self-awareness is how an individual consciously knows and understands their own character, feelings, motives, and desires. There are two broad categories of self-awareness: internal self-awareness and external self-awareness.[107]
- Consciousness refers to your individual awareness of your unique thoughts, memories, feelings, sensations, and environment. Essentially, your consciousness is your awareness of yourself and the world around you. This awareness is subjective and unique to you. If you can describe

[104] "Awareness," en.wikipedia.org/wiki/Awareness.
[105] "Awareness," Cambridge International Dictionary of English, 6th ed.
[106] K. Cherry, "What is Consciousness?" https://www.verywellmind.com/what-is-comsciousness-2795922#:-:text=Consciousness refers to your individual,feelings%2 sensations%2C and en.
[107] "Self-Awareness," en.wikipedia.org/wiki/Self-Awareness.

something you are experiencing in words, it is part of your consciousness.[108] Consciousness, or mind, is not matter. But even quantum mechanics is having a hard time describing consciousness.[109]

- Recollection (or recall) in memory refers to the mental process of retrieving information from the past. Along with encoding and storage, it is one of the three core processes of memory. There are three main types of recall: free recall, cued recall, and serial recall.[110]

Therefore, it is not merely the extension of physical life that is the ultimate goal, but rather the extension of our unique and individual awareness and consciousness.

The term *donor* may appear confusing since you may naturally assume that when referring to the human head being transplanted onto another body, it is the head that should be referred to as the donor. However, this is not the case. The head is referred to as the recipient, meaning it is receiving the donated body. Recipient is the head, with the body removed, so the body of the donor (corpse), with the head removed, can be donated to the supposedly living transferred head.

Extending physical life and awareness involves two different scientific endeavors. There are far greater limitations imposed upon extending human life than those involved with extending human awareness. The primary limiting factor involving the human body is the human body. No matter how many improvements or discoveries are incorporated to extend human life, there is an ultimate limit as to how long human flesh can remain productive and functional.

---

[108] K. Cherry, "What is Consciousness?"
[109] C. Sarich, "The Mind vs, Brain Debate (What is Consciousness?)" https://www.cuyamungueinstitute.com/article-and-news/the-mind-vs-brain-debate-what-is-consciousness.
[110] "Recall (memory)," en.wikipedia.org/wiki/Recall (memory).

3

Life Expectancy

Life expectancy is always defined statistically as the average number of years remaining at a given age. For example, a population's life expectancy at birth is the same as the average age at death for all people born in the same year.[111]

During the sixteenth century, Spanish explorer Ponce de Leon believed that a mythical and fabled spring, The Fountain of Youth, with its alleged ability to restore the youth of anyone who drinks or bathes in its waters could be found in what was to be the state of Florida. He sailed with Christopher Columbus in 1493 to the Americas during the second voyage of Columbus.[112] Since that time to the present, humanity has continued to seek the elusive Fountain of Youth through both legitimate, alleged, and fraudulent miracle drugs and other such remedies (i.e., the elixir for immortality).

In the spring of 2013, Pew Research conducted an opinion poll that found 38 percent of Americans would choose life extension treatments, while 56 percent would reject them.[113] The poll also determined that 63 percent of the public believed that efforts to prolong life were a good thing, 41 percent of Americans believed

---

[111] "Longevity," enwikipedia.org/wiki/Longevity.
[112] "Fountain of Youth," en.wikipedia.org/wiki/Fountain of Youth.
[113] "Life extension," en.wikipedia.org/wiki/Life extension.

that life extension would be good for society, and 51 percent believed it would be bad for society.[114]

Starting with a life expectancy reference point during the Bronze Age, the life expectancy at birth (LEB) was twenty-six years. In the year 2010, the world LEB was 67.2.[115] It's hard to conceive that life could be so short at that time; however, there was virtually no medical response to almost all illnesses and diseases or even accidents or injuries from warfare.

Mathematically, life expectancy is the mean number of years of life remaining at a given age.[116] The life expectancy of a woman is greater than that of a male. There are many reasons why a female lives longer. For example, men have historically consumed far greater amounts of tobacco, alcohol, and drugs than women do. Thus, they are more likely to die due to the related diseases like lung cancer, tuberculosis, and cirrhosis of the liver.

Men are also more likely today to die from unintentional injuries, (e.g., occupational hazards, war, or car accidents) or intentional causes (e.g., suicide).[117] In addition, men are more likely to die from other leading causes of death, including cancer of the respiratory system, emphysema, prostate cancer, and coronary heart disease. These far outweigh the female mortality rate from breast cancer and cervical cancer.[118] It has also been determined that women have more resistance to infections and degenerative diseases.[119]

Life expectancy has varied over the years for many reasons; however, the overall increase has evolved primarily due to dramatic improvements within the ever-expanding medical device and pharmaceutical industries involving significant advancements through their product research activities and formulation of new drugs. Moreover, dramatic advancements in medical treatment and

---

[114] Id.

[115] "Life expectancy," en.wikipedia.org/wiki/Life expectancy.

[116] Id.

[117] Id.

[118] Id.

[119] Id.

caring for various patient injuries, diseases, and diagnoses of vital organ problems and enhanced surgical procedures have greatly contributed to the extension of life. As indicated by the UN findings, the combined life expectancy for both men and women is expected to continue increasing for the foreseeable future.[120] The maximum human lifespan is currently speculated to be 115 years. The oldest recorded human, who lived to be 122, was Jeanne Calment, who died in 1997.[121]

Other scientists speculate the maximum life span to be 125 years.[122] However, there does not currently exist adequate advancements within the medical, pharmaceutical, or device industries or the scientific community to support a maximum life span of 125 years.[123]

There is also continued debate among scientists and others as to what is believed to be the furthest possible extent of human life. Professor Stuart Kim of Stanford University has speculated that in about 90 years, the first person at age 50 today will reach the age of 150 years. He has also asserted that he believes there are those alive today who will live to be 200 years old.[124]

While the potential ability for an individual to reach age 150 in about 90 years may be a reasonable expectation, based on the continued and dramatic advancements in all related fields, the belief that a person living today will reach an age of 200 years is an unrealistic and fanciful expectation. In order to accomplish such a dramatic increase in life expectancy over such a short period of time would require unrealistic achievements in many required support disciplines. Nonetheless, Professor Tom Kirkwood of Copenhagen and Newcastle University believes that there is no biological process

---

[120] Id.

[121] "Aging," en.wikipedia.org/wiki/Aging.

[122] "Life extension," enwikipedia.org/wiki/Life extension.

[123] Id.

[124] G. Taylor, "Scientist thinks the world's first 200-year-old person has already been born," https://norwaytoday.info/everyday/scientist-thinks-worlds-first-200-year-old-person-already-born.

that puts an absolute limit on maximum age.[125] However, there is currently no research data to support such exaggerated speculation.

Some researchers believe that in the future, humans will have indefinite life spans resulting from a total rejuvenation that will produce a healthy youthful condition. They speculate, with no estimation of when, that critical advancements in revitalizing tissue, stem cells, regenerative medicine, molecular repair, gene therapy, pharmaceutical, and organ replacement, including artificial organs, will enable an "indefinite life span."[126]

Such speculation is more than dubious and unrealistic because the human body that would house all these rejuvenated and replacement parts will eventually lack the viability to support their combined functions indefinitely. There would undoubtedly be a weak link in the process that would eventually result in the inability of the body and its living tissue to support the continuation of life, let alone an "indefinite life span."

However, while such future achievements in science, medicine, technology, and the medical industry may not provide humanity with endless life, it certainly is a reasonable expectation that human life extension would be dramatically prolonged. It should also be noted that the various methods that will eventually provide some amount of life extension to people beyond what is currently available will undoubtedly be accessible to only the privileged few with the financial resources and capability to pay the exorbitant cost for the products, systems, and surgical procedures to extend one's life.

Unless the government promulgates appropriate laws and regulations to assure accessibility to future life extension treatments and procedures to all, the availability of life extension opportunities will be relegated to only the very rich and privileged population.

With a greater understanding of the mechanisms that cause or contribute to the aging process and the subsequent advancements in medicine and related research discoveries, the prior boundaries

---

[125] Id.

[126] "Life Extension," en.wikipedia.org/wiki/Life extension.

of life expectancy will be extended dramatically. Nonetheless, there is a limit to which life expectancy can be extended. Eventually, even with the ability to replace all vital body parts (with the exception of the brain), including life-sustaining drugs and advanced therapeutic treatments, the existing flesh will eventually decline, deteriorate, and fail.

4

Is Achieving Immortality a Realistic or Worthy Expectation?

It depends upon who you ask. What would be your response? It is a realistic expectation that in the future, all diseases and other biologically contracted illnesses that terminate life will be curable or, more accurately stated, preventable. However, even if all life-terminating illnesses and diseases were eradicated, this eventuality remains a long distance from any reality that nears the definition of immorality. Again, in my opinion, there is no possibility of an immortal existence, rather just a lot of extended years.

One day in the future, people will undoubtedly look back and wonder how difficult and primitive life was for those of us living in an environment where humanity was so vulnerable and susceptible to a multiple of diseases and illnesses that were fatal in a manner as we today look back to the Middle Ages when civilization was exceptionally vulnerable to a multitude of diseases that no longer exist today or that can be effectively treated.

The leading cause of death in the future will involve those aspects of life that will remain unchanged, such as suicides, homicides, acts of war, and eventually the end of life through the aging process, no matter how long life is extended in the flesh. Simply put, flesh must eventually die.

There is no eternal existence for the human body or any of its components, even if continued organ transplants and other improvements to stabilize and maintain the body were implemented, including the successful transplant of the brain into an artificial realm of existence with specialized medications, stimulation, and modifications to the artificial housing. Eventually any and all human flesh will cease to exist.

According to Rosemberg, *Discourse on Immortality* bears a semantic difficulty concerning the word *death*. We usually define it in physiological terms as the cessation of biological functions that make life possible. But if immortality is the continuation of life after death, a contradiction appears to come up. Apparently it makes no sense to say that someone has died and yet survived death. To be immortal is precisely not to suffer death. Thus, whoever dies stops existing; nobody may exist after death, precisely because death means the end of existence.[127]

My perspective is somewhat different than Rosemberg's. As I stated previously, there cannot be life without awareness, with the acknowledgment that human existence can continue without awareness as it involves individuals who are comatose with their biological existence, dependent upon artificial respiration and drugs.

Immortality is not the continuation of life but rather the continuation of awareness. The term *life* cannot exist within the concept of an immortal existence, at least within the earthly realm. Death pertains to the living entity only; thus, there cannot be human life after death in the sense that death effectively terminates with our understanding of life.

For example, no matter how advanced artificial intelligence becomes in the future, especially as it pertains to an existing human awareness within an artificial housing, it cannot be referred to as something that is alive. Software and hardware can never produce nor be defined as something that is alive, other than in a metaphoric sense.

---

[127] G. Andrade, "Immortality," https://iep.utm.edu>immortality.

At the point in time when one has died and yet their awareness continues is not a contradiction, as discussed later, involving the death of the body while the brain continues to experience awareness. Death of the human body does not necessarily mean the end of existence since the focus of neuroscientists and other related disciplines has been to determine how our awareness, memories, and conscience can continue beyond the limitations imposed by the body, including the actual death of the body.

Such existence for future generations, free of the life-threatening health hazards that have pervaded our lives from the beginning of recorded history until today, will certainly extend life considerably, but not a life without an end. Every living organism has a biological clock, down to a single cell, with a self-established termination date, plus or minus a duration of time.

However, as discussed later, human awareness, absent the body and without physical life, may indeed reside on the fringes of continued unabated existence. Our human flesh will remain the anchor that stifles the freedom of our awareness to break free of its dependence upon the body, even if we are only referring to the brain in order to continue its existence.

Many religious groups believe immortality awaits their continued existence in the afterlife. However, our discussion relevant to an elusive immortality is not intended to involve the hereafter existence of our continued awareness as with the soul's awareness and existence after death. That is certainly a subject unto itself.

Rather, our entire focus is on life extension and longevity at various times during the evolution and advancements of medical scientists, neuroscientists, and other related research scientists and engineers who have dedicated their careers to understanding this subject. There is certainly a line in the sand between life on this side and nonlife, death involving the soul on the other side. Our focus will remain on this side of that line. Our discussion will follow the various achievements of medical scientists as they venture further and further into discovery and unlocking the critical answers to the extension of life in order to prolong human awareness.

However, let us assume for the moment that immortality is achievable. What would be the expectations of any individual if they were given the opportunity to experience immortality? What would be the anticipated reality, assuming the word *reality* would apply to immortality?

Most individuals would fantasize about a never-ending existence of youth with joyful bliss, happiness, adventure, and freedom from the burdens of their prior existence. Some would feel the relief of having escaped their fears and anticipation of their ultimate demise. Some individuals fear the prospect of death so intensely that they would pursue any option that would avail any possible hope of extending their life.

For example, many individuals have currently committed their physical body, or head, to the promise of cryopreserving their body until some future time when they can hypothetically be awakened to continue their life existence after a cure has been discovered for the cause of their death or potential death. These individuals would undoubtedly and enthusiastically accept the risks of achieving the remote possibility of immortality, or the further continuance of their life, as the ultimate answer to their quest. The subject of cryogenic preservation is discussed later.

Google co-founder Larry Page funded a start-up venture called Calico with the optimistic, although unrealistic and native, belief that his new venture could extend the human life span by a century and make good progress within reasonable timescales.[128] His optimism is based in part upon his employees, like Ray Kurzweil, a scientist and futurist employed by Google as a director of engineering who believes that if we can survive until the 2040s, we can live long enough to live forever. Kurzweil also believes that human beings will achieve immortality by fully merging with machines.[129]

Another start-up venture attempting to achieve immortality is the Methuselah Foundation, established by co-founder Aubrey de

---

[128] M. Shermaer, "Radical Life Extension Is Not Around the Corner," https://www. scientificamerican.com/article/radical-life-extension-is-not-around-the-corner.
[129] Id.

EDWARD W. REESE, PH.D.

Grey and funded by co-founder Peter Thiel. de Grey, a biomedical gerontologist, treats aging as an engineering problem to be solved at the cellular level by reprogramming cells to stop aging, or to live indefinitely. de Grey is on record claiming that the first human to live a thousand years is alive today.[130]

There is no living forever, no immortal existence regarding the human body. Obviously, Page and de Grey must have prepared a business plan for their new ventures. It would be interesting to determine how these scientists intend to accomplish such an enormous undertaking, especially within such optimistic scheduled objectives.

What Specific Reference to Immortality Am I Alluding To?

Again, remember that we are limiting our discussion about immortality to the world that does not include any regard to a spiritual afterlife. To further this discussion regarding immortality, let us assume that at some distant time in the future, scientists have indeed opened the door to immortality for human awareness and conscious to the extent that qualified candidates could apply for the transcending experience from their current existence into an unknown but anticipated immortal existence.

However, candidates in the distant future who would consider entering the unknown realm of immortality could not be advised as to what their forthcoming experience would involve because there is only, at best, speculation based upon the absence of sufficient empirical knowledge. There is simply no possibility to examine the supposedly immortal sphere in any manner at any time. The essence of immorality would forever elude the understanding of human thinking and may in fact represent another dimension entirely. We simply cannot know.

---

[130] Id.

Also, the process that would permit awareness to continue unabated is unknown. There has never been, and most likely will not be, any feedback as to the experiences of immortality. Will it have the capacity to exist with the total recovered memory of the individual during their physical life? Would there be unexpected boundaries that prohibit the transfer of certain human characteristics, such as emotions, curiosity, or the ability and desire to learn, that create unexpected boundaries that prohibit the transfer of certain human characteristics, such as emotions, curiosity, or the ability and desire to learn, within the realm of immortality? In other words, would the transcended you in an immortal existence be the same you, or would you become something less or different?

I speculate the unknown answer to this question would dissuade many potential candidates to seriously reconsider such eventuality. The potential downside could present a potential unspeakable dimension of horror from which the subject awareness could never escape.

There are, however, some definitive realities that are known. For example, the journey into an immortal existence would be a one-way trip. There is no coming back; nor is there any ability to communicate with the living world of humanity. Once the transfer into immortality occurs, continued awareness is forever captive within the realm of that unknown existence, be it heaven, hell, or something in between.

So will the immortal awareness have any ability to communicate with another immortal entity? Some scientists believe that telepathy would be a possible method for one mind to communicate with another mind, at least within the living world. Peter Hulsroj of Vienna, Austria, presents an interesting concept for the continuation of personality and consciousness, wherein he states,

On the consciousness level there are technically enabled possibilities of immortality as well. It might be possible to telepathically network consciousness between several individuals. Many individuals thus creating a pool of consciousness. When one of the individuals die the experiences of that individual will live on in the collective. Similarly, it may be possible to upload personalities.[131]

The reality of telepathic communication has been suggested as a possibility for many years, but never effectively demonstrated and certainly never validated as a means of communicating from one mind to another, absent the involvement of any human senses.

Science has thus far not identified any aspect of the human brain that could transmit a message to a receiving aspect of another's brain. Telepathy has typically been relegated to the mystical powers of the occult and has no significance within the realm of science. In the future, there may be a method of communicating from one mind to another via a process similar to a radio signal, for lack of a better term, that could be delivered and received by an implanted chip, or enhanced AI device. Telepathy is basically defined as the supposed process of communicating through means other than the human senses, such as direct exchange of human thoughts.[132]

Another related definition is *thought transference*, or transference of thought by extrasensory means from the mind of one individual to another.[133] For example, Alistair Jennings, PhD in neuroscience from University College London, has stated that the act of transferring thoughts into someone's head is now real.[134] Dr. Jennings believes we can read the electrical activity from brain cells with electronic devices and then transmit the signal, like we do the internet, and turn it back into brain cell activity.[135] However, Dr. Jennings also acknowledges some serious problems that remain unresolved, for example:

---

[131] P. Hulsroj, "What Is Immortality?" In *What If We Don't Die?* https://doi.org/10.1007/978-3-319-19093-8_17.

[132] "Telepathy," American Heritage Dictionary of the English Language, 5th ed.

[133] Id.

[134] A. Jennings, "Telepathy Is Real," https://www.facebook.com/Inside Science, p.2. https://insidescience.org/video/telepathy-real.

[135] Id.

- How exactly do you read brain activity?
- How do we decode the signals we've got?
- We actually still don't understand the brain codes electrical information.[136]
- How do we beam a thought back into someone else's head?[137]

As such, Dr. Jennings ultimately concluded that the technology to bring all those steps up to scratch for proper thought transmission still doesn't exist. And even if it did exist, we still need to work out how to understand the brain's language first.[138]

Therefore, if telepathy has not yet been achieved and, in my opinion, is not a realistic possibility involving living humans, it certainly cannot be a viable mechanism of awareness mobility within the immortal realm of continued existence. Moreover, even if telepathy were possible, there would not be any scientific ability to validate its efficacy within the realm of immortality. There is simply no method of retrieving data from an incorporeal (in or with the body) existence, if that is the reality of immortality.

Bernard Williams has argued that should life continue indefinitely, it would be terribly boring and therefore pointless. However, other philosophers counter that some activities may be endlessly repeated without ever becoming boring.[139] Even if some activities may be endlessly repeated without becoming boring, immortality would nonetheless eventually become boring and lonely. How could it not be when we consider that such an experience would literally continue forever without end? How much observation and information can be processed during an immortal existence without repetition?

Hulsroj further questions:

- What if personalities are uploaded to computers but not networked?

---

[136] Id.

[137] Id.

[138] Id.

[139] G. Andrade, "Immortality."

- Would that be human life as we know it and want it?
- What about the original self being left over in the moral coil?
- What if you make successive uploads?

Copies of the self would be made, but you would presumably remain corporally (in or with the body) bound.[140]

Would an Immortal Awareness Be Dynamic or Static?

It would logically appear, assuming logic can relate to immortality in any manner, that awareness existing within an immortal sense would be static with regards to its awareness location or position and incapable of any perceived movement.

The experience of awareness and consciousness would also appear to reside within a realm where there is no reality of location or the capability to move awareness from one location to another, again assuming there is any reality of location within an immortal existence.

If there were the possibility of mobile awareness within an immortal existence, the concerns for a boring or lonely existence would theoretically no longer be relevant. However, what aspect of mobility, external to any relationship with continued awareness, within an immortal existence, would be capable of movement involving awareness? These would be two independent entities. That is, the transferred human awareness into an immortal existence would not retain the ability to generate any movement any more than an individual could initiate their movement from place to place by simply thinking about it.

For example, if a mobile immortal existence were possible, could such awareness travel throughout the world, or for that matter, could it travel to other planets? It sounds crazy, I know, but such would be

---

[140] P. Hulsroj, "What Is Immortality If We Don't Die?"

the realm of the unknown immorality if there were the possibility of a continued awareness becoming a mobile existence.

Moreover, would the realm of awareness constitute a unique position where only one awareness and conscience can reside? If there are other awareness entities in existence, are they all separated from each other? Or does all awareness share the same unorthodox dimension? Within the same inexplicable realm of immortality, can one awareness communicate with another awareness or many other such entities?

Here again, if an individual awareness can communicate with another awareness or other such beings, the potential concern of being bored or lonely would assumedly no longer apply. However, again another dilemma arises. With what mechanism would the individual awareness residing within an immortal existence transmit and/or receive communications with other entities? Therefore, it would appear that no tangible asset would be available to cause the movement of awareness.

In Paul Edward's words, "So far from living on in paradise, a person deprived of his body and thus of all human sense organs would, quite aside from many other gruesome deprivations, be in a state of desolate loneliness and eventually come to prefer annihilation."[141]

If immortality would one day become a reality, and again I certainly believe it will not, I would consider it a bridge far too far, to state the very least. Immortality would be the continued, never-ending existence of awareness without any control or opportunity for changing any aspect of one's awareness. There would simply be the awareness that you exist in some forever unknown experience.

Furthermore, in the distant future when immortality would supposedly be achievable, in keeping with the optimistic scientific narrative, what would be the stature of awareness? It would undoubtedly not constitute any human flesh or brain since science would have evolved the continued awareness process to highly

---

[141] G. Andrade, "Immortality."

elaborate and very sophisticated housings, such as humanoids, or, more likely, even well beyond these structures.

Therefore, the mechanism or entity that would retain awareness would most likely not represent any living being but rather a computer or other data retrieval and storing capability that would retain the awareness and memory of a once-living person or perhaps some other method of mind storage and retrieval long separated from any human existence, including the brain. This topic is discussed in greater detail later in this book.

With the remote possibility of achieving immortality, I do not believe that immortality, within the confines discussed herein, can be achieved, although it appears probable that one day science may very well be close to looking into the abyss of immortality and, by curiosity, be tempted to open pandora's box.

As such, scientists will continue to unveil the secrets and mysteries of the human body and the brain and become more optimistic about the future longevity of human awareness. Such advances provide greater justification that in the future, albeit distant future, humanity may very well experience their continued existence and awareness to near the level of immortality, but never in an actual state of immortality, just very long life spans.

I believe that anything created by man cannot accomplish immortality, considering the full understanding of what is meant by the term *immortality* (never-ending). For example, would the immortal awareness of an entity continue unabated for a thousand years, a million years, or a billion years? I think not.

Moreover, humanity is incapable of achieving perfection in any of its creations, no matter how advanced it becomes. Even within greatly advanced humanoid robots, there would ultimately be a failure resulting in the termination of the entity. Perfection, at best, is only a momentary thing and certainly not forever.

However, the goal to accomplish perfection, as the term implies in all endeavors, is certainly worthy of enormous effort, especially within the science that advances life and benefits humanity, even though pure eternal perfection can never be achieved.

Nonetheless, after having presented such a dismal expectation for any realistic possibility of human immortality, one very far-reaching concept could accomplish true immortality. This distant future arrival at life everlasting requires not only discarding the human body but also any artificially entity that houses awareness. This future speculative accomplishment for the eternal existence of awareness is discussed later in this review.

Three Phases of Extending Life

We will investigate three phases of life and/or awareness extension involving current endeavors, near-future progress, and far future endeavors.

How Do We Currently Extend Life?

Within our current culture, we inhibit life's natural process toward our ultimate demise by life-sustaining drugs and artificial methods of life extension by machines that prolong life, even if our cognitive abilities are no longer fully functional.

We place our comatose loved ones in hospitals and nursing homes, often with a multitude of wires and equipment attached to keep their body functioning when the ones we remember and loved are no longer aware of our presence. Nursing homes are filled with the elderly who require constant monitoring and attention to their personal needs, many lacking self-dignity and loss of independence. They deteriorate until the point where they are placed in hospice care, usually unaware that their death is near.

This is certainly not the extended life that is the subject of this discussion. This is something else that lacks in any manner the benefits of extending one's life. Under these conditions, the elderly are simply being maintained and housed, which is the reality of our times.

The current realities of extending life by draconian efforts is the reverse of what it should be. In other words, life is worthy of extending and prolonging its awareness only if the result produces a life worth living without the typical discomforts and pains suffered during the elder years. Therefore, the prerequisite to prolonging someone's life must be accompanied with the individual's awareness, well-being, dignity, and independence fully intact.

As such, the exponential advances in medical and scientific research to extend life are outpacing similar advancements that address the aging problem. These two emphases must be amalgamated into a consolidated effort targeted at accomplishing life extension that would warrant the effort.

5

Free Antiaging and Life Extension Available to All

Since the narrative focus of this journey is the understanding of human life longevity and the continued existence of awareness, then perhaps the most logical starting point would pertain to taking personal inventory of circumstances in your life that limit both issues. In other words, let's start with the right here and right now of the current physical and emotional status of your well-being and the specific health hazards not conducive to extending your life.

Certainly not all factors that affect our health, longevity, and aging can be controlled. However, many life factors can be changed, or at least modified, although such corrective measures are often exceedingly difficult, demanding sacrifice, commitment, and continual monitoring.

Following is a discussion of potential common hazardous lifestyles that are self-imposed and consequently shorten life expectancy and awareness of the offender, at times to a significant extent. The discussion of hazardous and life-shortening habits and activities will sound punitive, harsh, and admonishing the reader, which is certainly not the intent. However, if you are sincere about wanting to understand the reality of factors that shorten or extend your life,

I encourage you to read the following with an honest interpretation as to your personal experience regarding each topic.

Tanning: An Avoidable Hazard to Life Longevity

Ironically, one of the most hazardous and potentially life-threatening premature aging circumstances involves sun tanning. The premature and permanent damage to the human skin is the direct result of unprotected, or overexposure, to UV sun radiation.

The ultimate damage caused by UV radiation exposure on the skin may not be apparent until many years later when it will eventually be witnessed as leathered, wrinkled skin and dark spots. At some future date, you may notice a difference between your skin and perhaps a friend or family member who did not tan and avoided overexposure to the sun's hazardous rays. Then it should become apparent that your days at the beach have finally rendered the ultimate consequence of your exposure to the sun and its destructive UV radiation. It is an obvious fact that those who tried to avoid the hazards of continued overexposure to the sun look and are perceived to be younger and healthier-looking than their age portrays.

UV radiation delivered by the sun will permanently damage cells in the epidermis, the outermost layer of the skin.[142] When skin damage occurs, it is a one-way process. There is no turning back.

What Happens When One Is Overexposed to UV Radiation

You go to the beach on a beautiful summer day and lay your blanket down on the sand, looking forward to achieving the ultimate healthy-looking tan, or so you and the masses who also flock to the beach perceive. Then through either lack of knowledge, ambivalence,

---

[142] "Epidermis," Medical Dictionary, 27th ed.

or simply not caring, you expose yourself to the sun's hazardous and potentially-deadly UV radiation.

The sun affects two layers of skin. The outer layer is the epidermis; the inner layer is the dermis. The outer epidermis layer contains a pigment called melanin, which acts like a dye. This pigment represents the body's attempt to defend itself against UV radiation. During this defensive process, the outer layer of skin results in a tan. In essence, a tan should provide a warning that the skin is in the process of producing irreversible and hazardous damage to the skin, including potential cancer. The damage to the skin caused by overexposure to the sun's UV radiation is accumulative and builds up over time with continued exposure to the sun. The inner layer of skin is called the dermis, where nerves and blood vessels are located.[143]

While sunbathers focus on their perceived healthy outer layer tan, they do not realize the damage that has been and continues to be occurring to the dermis second layer of skin. Here is where the sun has penetrated the skin cells, causing significant skin damage.

As the melanin is attempting to protect your skin, it will continue to elicit a darker and darker-colored skin tan with continued exposure to the sun's UV radiation. The sunbather perceives the opposite message indicated by the darker shade of skin tan, as the longer I remain in the sun, the more attractive my temporary tan will be, not realizing the irreversible damage taking place in both layers of their skin.

I have spoken with many people, especially teenagers and young adults, for many years about the serious hazards and even potential deadly consequences that can result from overexposure to the sun's UV radiation. Most teenagers and many younger adults seem oblivious to the serious hazards associated with exposure to the sun's UV rays. They tend to believe that a tan is attractive and even healthy. However, there is no such thing as a healthy tan. There is no health-redeeming aspect to exposing oneself to prolonged hazardous UV radiation produced by the sun.

---

[143] "Effects of Sun Exposure," https://familydoctor.org/effects-early-sun-exposure.

The price to be paid for a perceived healthy tan, especially at a young age, that lasts only a few days will become a disappointing reminder in later years as the permanent effects appear more and more evident in the mirror, potentially resulting in skin cancer. This inevitable result could have been avoided if those who tend to worship the sun at any age recognized the reality of exposing oneself to the dangers of UV radiation.

The younger you start tanning and the more you tan, the greater the risk of acquiring premature aging of the skin and possibly skin cancer.

There Is No Such Thing as a Safe Tan!

There are three types of ultraviolet rays emitted from the sun, all having powerful properties that produce sunburn and tanning action in the skin, but each type affects the skin differently. UVA rays come from the sun and can cause premature skin aging, wrinkling, and skin cancer. UVA radiation also comes from sun lamps and tanning beds. It may also cause problems with the eyes and the immune system.[144] UVB radiation causes sunburn, darkening and thickening of the outer layer of the skin, melanoma, and other types of skin cancer.[145] UVC rays are the most dangerous; however, they offer little threat since these rays cannot penetrate the earth's protective ozone layer.[146]

Following are some of the serious premature aging side effects associated with overexposure to the sun's UV radiation.

There are two main types of skin cancer: melanoma and non-melanoma. Melanoma is the less common but more dangerous type of skin cancer and is responsible for the majority of deaths every year.

---

[144] "UVA Radiation," https:///www.cancer.gov/publications/dictionaries/cancer-terms/def/uva-radiation.

[145] "UVB radiation," https:///www.cancer.gov/publications/dictionaries/cancer-terms/def/uvb-radiation.

[146] "UVC radiation," https:///www.cancer.gov/publications/dictionaries/cancer-terms/def/uvc-radiation.

This form of skin cancer begins in the epidermal cells where melanin is produced. According to the American Cancer Society, melanoma is almost always curable when detected in its early stages.[147] Non-melanomas will typically form on the body areas exposed to the cells that make pigment.[148]

Other Skin Changes

A clump can form in some skin cells with melanin, creating freckles and moles that can eventually become cancer.[149]

Eye Damage

Clouding of the natural lens of the eye causing decreased vision and possible blindness are all effects of cataracts. Studies have indicated that this form of eye damage could result from increased exposure to UV radiation.[150]

Moreover, just one day in the sun without proper eye protection, like sunglasses, may result in a burned cornea, the outer, clear membrane layer of the eye.[151] The best way to protect your eyes is to wear sunglasses that provide 100 percent UV protection.

Lowered Immune System

When UV radiation burns the skin, white blood cells can produce new cells; however, doing so can put the immune system at risk in other areas.[152]

---

[147] "The Risk of Tanning," U.S. Food & Drug Administration (FDA), April 26, 2019.
[148] Id.
[149] "Effects of Sun Exposure," https://familydoctor.org/effects-early-sun-exposure.
[150] "The Risk of Tanning," U.S. Food & Drug Administration (FDA), April 26, 2019.
[151] "Cornea," The American Heritage Dictionary, Second College Edition.
[152] "The Hard Truth About Tanning," Impact Melanoma, info@impactmelanoma.org.

Sunburn

Sunburn is a serious step up from tanning. It occurs when the skin is unable to produce enough melanin quick enough to prevent UV radiation from damaging the surface of the skin and the blood vessels located deeper in the second layer of the skin.[153]

Sunburn will turn the surface layer of the skin red and elicit significant pain caused by damage to these blood vessels, including inflammation and swelling. Severe sunburn can cause enough inflammation that people become nauseated and sick. It can take up to forty-eight hours to see the full effect of sunburn.[154] Just one bad sunburn can more than double the chances of developing skin cancer.[155]

Tanning Beds: Another Avoidable Hazard to Life Longevity

Those who like tanning tend to establish or maintain their tan throughout the year by artificial methods involving the use of tanning beds, especially at times when natural tanning from the sun is not available or inconvenient. Tanning salons are in many strip malls and very popular, especially among young Caucasian girls who comprise the largest group. 2.5 million teenagers use tanning beds each year, including 35 percent of girls aged seventeen, with many as young as thirteen.[156]

The American Academy of Dermatology has determined that 63 percent of teenagers believe they look better with a tan. Moreover,

[153] "Dangers of Outdoor Tanning," https://www.aimatmelanoma.org/prevention/dangers-of-tanning-and-burning.
[154] Id.
[155] "Tanning Bed vs. Sun Rays: Which is More Dangerous" https://www.unitypoint.org/livewell/article.aspx?id=93cb5a65-b789-43ce-b3f7-4d57572e8ca0.
[156] "The Dangers of Tanning Beds," https://familydoctor.org/the-dangers-of-tanning-beds.

they report that 28 percent of female teens and 14 percent of male teens claim they never use any tanning lotion to protect their skin.[157]

Ironically, these tanners are spending money to continue the process of destroying their skin through the use of tanning beds, apparently unaware or not troubled with the reality that the use of tanning beds is carcinogenic to humans. In 2009, the World Health Organization's International Agency for Research on Cancer classified UV tanning beds as Class 1 human carcinogens. Class 1 is the highest risk category.[158] Those who use tanning beds are at much greater risk of developing cancer. It is estimated that the risk of cancer increases by about 75 percent for those who use tanning beds before the age of thirty-five.[159]

Some promoters of tanning bed use claim that indoor tanning is a far more effective method of obtaining a superior tan. They also push indoor tanning as healthy because it provides the body with a source of vitamin D. However, these sales claims are inaccurate and falsely promote a positive outcome with the use of tanning beds **that emit approximately twelve times more UV radiation than natural sunlight** (emphasis added).[160] There simply is nothing healthy or advantageous about tanning either indoors or on a beach. For example, using a tanning bed for twenty minutes is equivalent to spending one to three hours a day at the beach with no sun protection at all. Tanning beds emit three to six times the amount of radiation given off by the sun.[161]

I have investigated cases where users of tanning beds have been subjected to profoundly serious burns from tanning beds. Photographs of these individual burn injuries would certainly motivate those who

---

[157] "The Hard Truth About Tanning," Impact Melanoma, info@impactmelanoma.org.
[158] "The Dangers of Tanning Beds," https://familydoctor.org/the-dangers-of-tanning-beds.
[159] Id.
[160] "Tanning Bed vs. Sun Rays: Which is More Dangerous?" https://www.unitypoint.org/livewell/article.aspx?id=93cb5a65-b789-43ce-b3f7-4d57572e8 ca0.
[161] "The Hard Truth About Tanning," Impact Melanoma, info@impactmelanoma.org.

use indoor tanning to reconsider the serious potential injuries they are exposing themselves to.

Vitamin D is essential for your health; however, it only takes five to ten minutes of unprotected sun two to three times a week to have the skin produce adequate amounts of this essential vitamin. Any amount of additional sun beyond this will not increase your vitamin D level but increase the risk of skin cancer.[162] It is far safer not to depend on exposure to the sun's UV radiation for vitamin D, but instead to obtain the recommended amount of vitamin D through daily supplements or drinks and foods that provide this vitamin.

In my opinion, the FDA and/or other appropriate governing agencies should make tanning beds illegal for their intended use since there is a significant lack of understanding or acceptance of the serious hazards associated with indoor tanning, especially as it pertains to young girls, coupled with the strong scientific findings that UV radiation produced by tanning beds clearly pose a serious threat that should be eliminated.

A purposed intent to obtain a tan, either by direct exposure to the sun's UV rays or artificially through the use of tanning beds, will certainly accelerate the irreversible and accumulative damage to the surface of your skin and deeper layers of tissue as well. For many, it will not become apparent until later in life, adding the physical appearance of extra years when their skin presents the result of tanning with premature aging.

Smoking: Another Avoidable Hazard to Life Longevity

As with the avoidable, self-imposed hazards associated with the sun's UV radiation, smoking is also a profoundly serious self-imposed hazard to the length of life. Smoking has caused seven of every ten cases of lung cancer. Other forms of cancer that affect other body

---

[162] "Tanning Bed vs. Sun Rays: Which is More Dangerous?" https://www.unitypoint.org/livewell/article.aspx?id=93cb5a65-b789-43ce-b3f7-4d57572e8 ca0.

parts due to smoking including the mouth, throat, voice box (larynx), esophagus (the tube between your mouth and stomach), bladder, bowel, cervix, kidney, liver, stomach, pancreas, and coronary heart disease.[163]

Smoking will also damage your heart and blood circulation and increase the risk of developing conditions such as heart attack, stroke, peripheral vascular disease (damaged blood vessels), and cerebrovascular disease (damage arteries that supply blood to the brain).[164] Moreover, smoking will also damage your lungs, leading to chronic obstructive pulmonary disease (COPD), obstructive-pulmonary-disease, emphysema, pneumonia, respiratory conditions (e.g., asthma), impotence, and reduced fertility (in both men and women).[165]

The toxins in cigarette smoke expose your skin to an oxidative (to combine or cause to combine with oxygen) stress.[166] This causes dryness, wrinkles, and other signs of premature aging.[167] Therefore, smoking is a profoundly serious and debilitating habit that clearly shortens a smoker's life span and reduces the quality of their life.

Those individuals who have unfortunately become addicted to smoking will not easily give up their craving for nicotine. Most smokers will not perceive the slow, damaging encroachment to their bodily functions caused by their smoking habit upon their vital organs, especially their lungs and respiratory system, until the symptoms obligate them to seek medical attention. For many, it will be too late.

Most smokers will not perceive the symptoms that obligate them to seek medical attention. For many, it will be too late. Even then, some smokers will continue to smoke regardless of the consequence

---

[163] "What are the health risks of smoking?" https:/www.nhs.uk/common-health-questions/lifestyle/what-are-the-health-risks-of-smoking.

[164] Id.

[165] Id.

[166] "Oxidize," Medical Dictionary, 27th ed.

[167] K. Watson, "Everything You Need to Know About Premature Aging," https://www.healthline.com/health/beauth-skin-care/premature-aging#tips-for-prevention.

to their health and life as their habit holds them prisoner without the apparent ability to escape. I have viewed the effects of a prolific smoker's lungs in a pathology lab. It is a frightening sight where the lung is difficult to recognize with a tarlike appearance on the surface

The overwhelming scientific evidence has validated the profoundly serious health hazards associated with smoking; thus the use of tobacco should have been forcibly removed by the FDA from public access many years ago. However, strong lobby groups for the tobacco industry have been successful in their protection from governmental intervention because of the wealth and influence of this industry. In addition, if an attempt were made by the FDA or another governmental agency to prohibit tobacco availability to the public, there would be such a social upheaval in protest that the attempt would undoubtedly fail in a dramatic manner, as did prohibition in the 1920s and 1930s.

Lastly on this subject, I appeal to you, the reader, with the strongest possible recommendation that if you smoke, consider the profound consequences to your health and longevity as described above. I realize that you did not purchase this book to receive a lecture on the hazards of smoking, but since I present a focused discussion on extending life, I cannot avoid a minimal discussion about this avoidable self-imposed hazard as well as other potential hazards discussed within this section.

Alcohol: Another Avoidable Hazard to Life Longevity

Drinking too much alcohol can harm your health. Excessive alcohol use led to 88,000 deaths and 2.5 million years of potential life lost each year in the United States from 2006 to 2010, shortening the lives of those who died by an average of thirty years. Further, excessive drinking was responsible for one in ten deaths among working-age adults aged twenty to sixty-four years.[168]

---

[168] "Alcohol Use and Your Health," https://www.cdc.gov/alcohol/fact-sheets/alcohol-use.ht.

The impact upon the human body starts with the first sip of alcohol. An occasional drink is not a concern. However, the continued and excessive drinking of alcoholic beverages will create serious health problems. Following are some health hazards and effects that alcohol use can cause: shrinking brain, blackouts, dependence, behavior changes, hallucinations, slurred speech, liver damage, pancreatitis, frequent diarrhea, infertility, sexual dysfunction, malnutrition, diabetic complications, numbness, lung infections, fatigue, stomach distress, birth defects, changes in coordination, and muscle cramps.[169]

The cumulative effects of excessive alcohol use can further result in the following health-related problems: digestive and endocrine glands, inflammatory damage, sugar level problems, circulatory system, sexual and reproductive health, skeletal and muscle system, immune system, night sweats, and alcohol allergies.[170]

Alcohol poisoning can happen when you drink a lot of alcohol in a brief period of time. This can cause the alcohol in your bloodstream to interfere with parts of your brain responsible for basic life support functions, such as breathing, body temperature, and heart rate. Left untreated, alcohol poisoning can cause permanent brain damage and death.[171]

Drinking alcohol excessively dehydrates your body. Over time, this dehydration can cause your skin to sag and lose its shape.[172] Alcoholic consumption is associated with the destruction of the nerve cells, which are responsible for memory encoding, storage, and retrieval.[173]

---

[169] A. Pietrangelo et al., "The Effects of Alcohol on Your Body," https://www.healthline.com/health/alcohol/effects-on-body#4.

[170] Id.

[171] A. Santos-Longhurst, "Does Alcohol Kill Brain Cells?" https://www.healthline/does-alcohol-kill-cells#brain-development.

[172] K. Watson, "Everything You Need to Know About Premature Aging," https://www.healthline.com/health/beauty-skin-care/premature-aging#tips-for-prevention

[173] "Long-Term Memory," Effects of Alcohol on Long-Term Memory.

Obesity: Another Avoidable Hazard to Life Longevity

More than a third of Americans are considered obese. The term means that an individual weighs more than 20 percent the weight that they should weigh above their ideal weight. Here again, for most obese persons, it's a self-imposed serious health hazard that shortens life expectancy, sometimes dramatically.

If you are in the category of an overweight individual, and especially if you are considered obese, you are subject to many serious health hazards, such as all-causes of death (mortality), high blood pressure (hypertension), high LDL cholesterol, low HDL cholesterol, elevated levels of triglycerides, type 2 diabetes, coronary heart disease, stroke, gallbladder disease, osteoarthritis (a breakdown of cartilage and bone within a joint), sleep apnea and breathing problems, many types of cancer, low quality of life, mental illness such as clinical depression, anxiety, and other mental disorders, body pain and difficulty with physical functioning.[174]

Inactive Lifestyle: Another Avoidable Hazard to Life Longevity

An inactive lifestyle is defined as an individual who spends a lot of time sitting and lying down with little or no exercise. Throughout the world, the tendency is toward spending increased time involved with sedentary activities.

It appears that humanity can be divided into two groups relevant to an active or inactive lifestyle. There are those who are actively involved in a scheduled routine of exercise or at least aware of the need to exercise to improve their overall health, for example, these individuals we see in the gyms and health clubs or wearing their bicycle clothes and helmets. Many individuals have active exercise programs at their home using various exercise equipment. Then

---

[174] "The Health Effects of Overweight and Obesity," Centers for Disease Control and Prevention (CDC).

there are the couch potato types who have little or no concern about exercise. They simply put on the pounds and live a tired and sluggish lifestyle.

If you are living an inactive lifestyle, you burn fewer calories. This makes you more likely to gain weight. You may lose muscle strength and endurance because you are not using your muscles as much. Your bones may get weaker and lose some mineral content. Your metabolism may be affected, and your body may have more trouble breaking down fats and sugars. Your immune system may not work as well. You may have poorer blood circulation. Your body may have more inflammation. You may develop a hormonal imbalance.[175]

The health risks to living an inactive lifestyle also include obesity, heart diseases, high blood pressure, high cholesterol, stroke, metabolic syndrome, type 2 diabetes, certain cancers including colon, breast, and uterine, osteoporosis and falls, and increased feelings of depression and anxiety.[176] Having a sedentary lifestyle can also raise your risk of premature death, and the more sedentary you are, the higher your health risks are.[177] People who practice physical exercise at moderate to elevated levels have a longer life expectancy compared to those who are not physically active. Moderate exercise has also been determined to result in a higher quality of life by reducing inflammation.[178]

The U.S. Department of Health and Human Services has concluded that these data very strongly supports an inverse association between lifetime physical activity and all-cause mortality with lifetime inactive individuals having a 30 percent higher risk of dying compared with lifetime active individuals. Thus, multiple

---

[175] "Health Risk of an Inactive Lifestyle," https://medlineplus.gov/healthrisksofaninactivelifestyle.html.
[176] Id.
[177] "Aging," en.wikipedia.org/wiki/Aging.
[178] Id.

epidemiological reports suggest that lifetime physical inactivity decreases average life expectancy.[179]

Therefore, as with the other avoidable hazards to life longevity discussed above, lack of regular exercise is certainly another self-imposed hazard to extending life.

Illegal Drugs: Another Avoidable Hazard to Life Longevity

Suffice it to say, and without belaboring the negative consequences of illegal drug use, thousands of people die every year from a drug overdose. Those who are victims and enslaved to various highly addictive drugs are not considering the serious, life-threatening consequences of their drug addiction. Nonetheless, the significant adverse effects on such a large population of Americans must be noted as a contributing factor in the loss of a normal life span and certainly without any consideration to extending their life.

The more predominate illegal drugs that cause so much pain, suffering, and death include methamphetamine, cocaine, ecstasy, and heroin.

Stress and Anxiety: Another Avoidable Hazard to Life Longevity

We all know what stress is. Most of us experience stress every day in one form or another and at various levels of intensity dependent upon our individual ability to process stressful situations. Stress is typically your emotional response to challenges or demands that place you outside your comfort zone.

A particular stressful situation may not elicit any emotional response from one person, while under the same circumstance, another person may rise to the level of rage. We are all unique as to

---

[179] F. Booth et al., "Lifetime sedentary living accelerates some aspects of secondary aging," https://journals.physiology.org/doi/full/10.1152/japplphysiol.00420.2011.

how we respond to various stressful circumstances based upon how we historically processed stressful situations from our early childhood.

Elevated stress levels experienced on a regular basis is a prerequisite for a hazardous health event to occur, including strokes, heart attacks, and premature death. Living with continual elevated stress is certainly not the life that anyone should be subjected to. If your stress level is continually high, it is like pressing the pedal in your car to the floor and keeping the tachometer in the red. Even if you have a high-performance vehicle (i.e., you're in top physical condition), your engine will eventually fail (i.e., die), as will any individual living a similar lifestyle.

The cause(s) of stress are typically easy to identify. What preoccupies your mind when driving to or from work, and how preoccupied are you? Does your particular stress problem(s) distract you to the point where your relationships are being affected? Or are you experiencing health-related problems directly related to your elevated stress level? Some individuals experience such elevated levels of focused stress that they may actually become disoriented and lose their awareness of where they are and the activity with which they are involved. They can become momentarily oblivious to their surroundings and the activity they were performing. Such momentary cognitive paralysis can be so debilitating that individuals have actually lost their lives by, for example, driving through a stop sign or a red light or other such hazardous situations.

Many factors and life experiences have influenced our specific mode of emotional and physical responses to stressful situations. The issue of how stress affects your health and longevity is relevant here because recurring and prolonged stress will produce serious health problems that can shorten one's life.

Stress takes us out of our comfort zone and into a realm of uncertainty, often based on a fear of an unknown outcome or consequence. Our individual insecurities picked up through our prior life experiences contribute to the stress and anxiety that we subsequently encounter and the manner as to how we process and react when these insecurities confront us.

Compare your own potential stress risk factors to the following lists of adverse health consequences that arise from continued exposure to your particular stress issues: headaches, heartburn, rapid breathing, risk of heart attack, increased depression, insomnia, weakened immune system, high blood sugar, high blood pressure, fertility problems, erectile dysfunction, missed periods, stomachache, low sex drive, and tense muscles.[180]

Additional common signs of stress include changes in mood, clammy or sweaty palms, diarrhea, difficulty sleeping, dizziness, anxiety, frequent sickness, grinding teeth, low energy, racing heartbeat, and trembling.[181] As a result, frequent or chronic stress will make your heart work too hard for too long. When your blood pressure rises, so do your risks for having a stroke or heart attack.

Anxiety is the mind and body's reaction to stressful, dangerous, or unfamiliar situations. It is the sense of uneasiness, distress, or dread you feel before a significant event.[182] Anxiety is not the same as stress and can produce serious and debilitating physical health hazards. Anxiety is your body's emotional response to stressful or hazardous situations that one may encounter, such as the dread or anticipation of bodily harm that a soldier may experience in combat.

While there are some similar characteristics to stressful conditions, anxiety produces its own list of potential health hazards, such as a sense of doom, depression, pounding heart, loss of libido, extreme fatigue, panic attacks, headaches, irritability, breathing problems, upset stomach, muscle aches, and other pains.[183]

The key point here to be emphasized regarding stress and anxiety is for you to recognize how potentially hazardous stress and anxiety may be affecting your life pertaining to both your physical and mental well-being. Moreover, these emotional and physically hazardous conditions, like the other avoidable hazards to your normal life span

---

[180] A. Pietrangelo, "The Effects of Stress on Your Body," https://www.healthline.com/health/stress/effects-on-body.
[181] E. Scott, "What Is Stress," https://www.verywellmind.com/stress-and-health-3145086.
[182] T. Jovanovic, "What is Anxiety?" https://www.anxiety.org/what-is-anxiety.
[183] "Sleep Deprivation," en.wikipedia.org/wiki/sleep deprivation.

as discussed previously, are potentially hazardous conditions that you should attempt to overcome or at least attempt to reduce the potential effects of these hazardous consequences to your health and your longevity. But make no mistake: living with elevated and continued stress and anxiety in your life will eventually take its toll and shorten your life expectancy, perhaps to a significant extent.

Sleep Deprivation: Another Avoidable Hazard to Life Longevity

Sleep deprivation involves many more profound consequences than feeling tired and fatigued in the morning and during the day. Failure to obtain an adequate night's sleep can result in serious current and long-term health consequences, including aching muscles, confusion, memory lapse or loss, depression, development of false memory, hand tremor, headaches, malaise, bags under the eyes, increased blood pressure, increased stress hormone levels, increased risk of type 2 diabetes, lowering of immunity (increased susceptibility to illness), increased risk of fibromyalgia, irritability, rapid involuntary rhythmic eye movement, obesity, seizure, violent behavior, yawning, and mania.[184]

Study after study has revealed that people who sleep poorly are at greater risk for a number of diseases and health problems. Sleep is vital for learning and memory, and lack of sleep impacts our health, safety, and longevity. Life expectancy is also dependent upon the amount and quality of sleep one receives.

Those who sleep longer, for six to seven hours every night, live longer. Those who sleep less than five hours each night more than double their risk of death from cardiovascular disease; however, those who sleep more than nine hours tend to double the risk of death, but not necessarily from cardiovascular disease.[185]

---

[184] "Consequences of Insufficient Sleep," healthysleep.med.harvard.edu/healthy/matters/consequences.
[185] Mayo Clinic, "Sleep Apnea."

Do You Have Sleep Apnea?

Sleep apnea is a potentially serious disorder in which breathing repeatedly stops and starts. If you snore loudly and feel tired even after a full night's sleep, you might have sleep apnea. The main types of sleep apnea are obstructive sleep apnea, the more common form that occurs when throat muscles relax; central sleep apnea, which occurs when your brain doesn't send proper signals to the muscles that control breathing; and complex sleep apnea syndrome, also known as treatment-emergent central sleep apnea, which occurs when someone has both obstructive sleep apnea and central sleep apnea.[186]

The most common signs and symptoms of obstructive and center sleep apneas include loud snoring; episodes in which you stop breathing during sleep, which would be reported by another person; gasping for air during sleep; awakening with a dry mouth; morning headache; difficulty staying asleep (insomnia); excessive daytime sleepiness (hypersomnia); difficulty paying attention while awake; and irritability.[187]

Sleep apnea can contribute to serious health issues; therefore, if you suspect that you may be experiencing any of these systems, it is essential that you seek medical intervention at the earliest opportunity.

Coffee Drinking

In the not-too-distant past, coffee drinking was considered potentially hazardous to your health primarily due to its caffeine content. Therefore, drinking non-decaffeinated coffee would have appeared on the above list of another avoidable hazard to life longevity.

In order to avoid the perceived health hazard associated with drinking regular coffee, many coffee drinkers switched to decaffeinated coffee. However, research has determined that

---

[186] Id.
[187] Id.

non-decaffeinated coffee is actually not only safe to drink but also has some very beneficial attributes. For example, a recent study from Queen Mary University of London indicated that drinking as many as twenty-five cups each day of regular coffee did not appear to have an impact on arteries.[188]

David DiSalvo at *Forbes* reports that in recent years, studies have found that drinking coffee was associated with lower mortality, healthier lives, protection against diabetes and dementia, as well as improved memory. Vivian Manning-Schaffel at NBC News reports that "researchers believe that caffeine consumption is associated with living longer, while antioxidants in coffee might account for other health benefits associated with drinking coffee.[189]

On the other side of the coin, solvents, like benzene, are used to decaffeinate coffee. Even in small amounts, benzene can cause drowsiness, dizziness, and headaches, as well as eye, skin, and respiratory tract irritation. Over the long term and in high doses, benzene has been linked to cancer, blood disorders, and fetal development issues in pregnant women.[190]

Methylene chloride is also another controversial chemical found in coffee that is decaffeinated. When inhaled even in small doses, it can cause coughing, wheezing, and shortness of breath. At higher doses, it can cause headache, confusion, nausea, vomiting, dizziness, and fatigue and has been found to cause liver and lung cancer in animals.[191]

If consumers want to be sure that synthetic solvents weren't used to decaffeinate, they should look for the organic seal, says Charlotte Vallaeys, *Consumer Reports* senior policy analyst and food-labeling

---

[188] J. Daley, "New Study Shows Coffee-Even 25 Cups a Day of It-Isn't Bad for Your Heart," https://www.smithsonianmag.com/smart-news/new-study-shows-coffee-even-25-cups-day-isnt-bad-for-heart-180972336/#:-:text=David DiSalvo at For.

[189] Id.

[190] J. Calbernone, "Is Decaffeinated Coffee Bad for You?" https://www.consumerreports.org/coffee/is-decaffeinated-coffee-bad-for-you.

[191] Id.

expert. That seal prohibits not only pesticides but chemical solvents during processing too.[192]

Physical Examinations Can Be a Lifesaver

While the previous list identifies adverse and high-risk contributing factors that will shorten your life expectancy, other than coffee drinking, and should be avoided or diminished, another very serious circumstance is the cause of many thousands of avoidable Americans deaths every year. I am referring to the basic and essential necessity to have a regularly scheduled physical examination at least once a year if no other pervasive condition is evident.

Many individuals have an attitude that "if it isn't broke, don't fix it." That is, if they are not having any physical symptoms, there is no need to see a physician. Or even if they have a symptom, many individuals will choose to ride the symptom out, tough through it, or buck up.

Others retain a fear of having a checkup, believing they may get some bad news about their condition or experience some level of pain associated with the examination. Such fears can be so profound that in some cases, they emotionally paralyze the person from reacting appropriately and seeking proper help.

I am aware of individuals who had such a dreadful fear of being vaccinated, regardless of the benefits that the shot would provide, that they refused to be inoculated. Perhaps the most common awareness of such fears involves the fear a child has, and many adults as well, to visiting a dental office.

Those who retain such fears are exceedingly apprehensive because they imagine the worst possible outcome and expect it to occur and therefore avoid visiting a physician, usually believing they will schedule an appointment sometime in the future.

Here's the real problem: during my many years as a forensic examiner, I have unfortunately encountered individuals who, for

---

[192] Id.

whatever their reluctance, refused to seek medical help for their condition and were subsequently informed by their health-care provider with words no one would ever want to hear, "If only you would have come to us sooner, we could have helped you."

Fear can be a killer. Therefore, I encourage you to schedule a yearly physical. I have a yearly physical at the Mayo Clinic, and when I leave the facility, I have a good feeling about the status of my health and the knowledge that I am aware of what issues need to be addressed, if any, with no lingering concerns (or fears of the unknown).

Should you have any persistent symptoms, I strongly urge you to schedule an appointment with your health-care provider who most often will assure you that your condition is not life-threatening and treat it appropriately. Don't let your hesitation possibly put you in a situation where you are told, "If only you would have come to us sooner, we could have helped you." Do it not just for yourself but also for those in your life who care about you.

Of course, I strongly recommend that you should schedule, at minimum, a through yearly exam before you encounter any potentially serious symptoms.

Other Aspects of Lifestyle That Affect Longevity

Certain diets, like the Mediterranean diet, have been found to lower the risk of heart disease and premature death. The major contributing factors to longevity relating to a diet include higher consumption of vegetables, fish, fruit, nuts, and monounsaturated fatty acids like olive oil.[193]

Loneliness and stress have a higher mortality risk than smoking. Effective stress-reducing factors include social activities, religious beliefs, and married life (especially for men), all of which contribute to longevity.[194] Of course, many other human diseases and body

---

[193] "Aging," en.wikipedia.org/wiki/aging.
[194] Id.

disorders result from the aging process that pose great risk to our continued life experience and to our ultimate death.

As medical intervention identifies and responds to each disease, defective organ, and system abnormality that threatens the well-being and longevity of life, these health hazards have been, and shall continue to be, identified and targeted for reduction or elimination through continued medical discovery and intervention. Yes, one day all known diseases today, including cancer, will no longer exist. Humanity will be virtually free of all such health hazards to human existence.

Conclusion on Avoidable Hazards to Life Longevity

I have discussed some of the major self-induced health hazards that will reduce, perhaps significantly, the possibility of extending the life expectancy of those involved. Specifically, I discussed the hazards of tanning and sunburn, smoking, alcohol, obesity, inactive lifestyle, illegal drugs, and stress and anxiety disorders while recognizing there are other factors as well.

If you are involved with any of the self-imposed health hazards discussed previously, especially if more than one is part of your lifestyle, you should recognize that you have chosen a lifestyle that is, without question, shortening your life expectancy to some extent and perhaps dramatically. In place of having self-imposed health hazards in your life, I encourage you to commit a strong focus on your activities, especially those listed above that can reduce the length of your life and well-being, and set your mind to reducing or limiting their hazardous effects.

Many of us have an attitude that we intend to deal with such health hazard problems in the near future. "Next week, I will start that diet, stop smoking or drinking, and so forth." However, it seems next week typically never comes. Often there is the legitimate and honest intent to correct what is known to be a hazardous habit or lifestyle that could ultimately and prematurely cause avoidable pain, suffering, and ultimate death.

And yet the immediate gratification, especially from addictions like smoking, alcohol, eating, and drugs, mask the price that will ultimately become due and payable. Waking up in the emergency room may provide a belated reality check of the consequence in failing to correct the avoidable lifestyle hazard, assuming one survives the emergency.

This discussion of hazardous and life-shortening habits and activities sounds punitive, harsh, and admonishing to the reader, which again is not the intent. A study conducted by Frank B. Hu, professor of nutrition and epidemiology at the Harvard T. H. Chan School, and others investigated five of the above potential hazards to lifestyle, including smoking, excessive alcohol consumption, physical inactivity, poor diet, and obesity, because an analysis of fifteen studies covering more than half a million people in seventeen nations had concluded that these unhealthy lifestyle factors could account for around 60 percent of premature deaths.[195]

Five Low-Risk Factors

The researchers calculated the extent to which early death was linked to the following five lifestyle-related low-risk factors: not smoking, moderate alcohol intake (in the region of up to one five-ounce glass of wine per day for women or two for men), regular exercise (or a half hour or more per day of moderate to vigorous activity), healthful diet (or being in the top 40 percent of a recognized healthful eating index), and normal weight (or having a body mass index [BMI] under 25).[196]

Bringing all the results together, the researchers produced nationally-representative estimates of longer life expectancy linked to each low-risk lifestyle factor and to all of them combined. They found that women who did not follow any of the five low-risk factors

---

[195] C. Paddock, "These five habits will lengthen your lifespan," https://www. medicalnewstoday.com/articles/321671#Life-expectancy-rises-with-each-factor.
[196] Id.

had a life expectancy of twenty-nine years at age fifty, compared with 43.1 years for those who adopted all five. There was a similar pattern for men, with those who did not adopt any of the five factors, having a life expectancy of 25.5 years at age 50, compared with 37.6 years for those who adopted all of them.[197]

Life expectancy at the time of birth in the United States rose from sixty-three years in 1940 to seventy-nine years in 2014.[198] The researchers suggest that without widespread obesity, this increase could have been much larger.[199] Today, it is commonly understood that obesity is the major contributing factor that affects mortality. Also R. Dale Hall and Andrew Peterson of the Society of Actuaries have identified nine factors that relate to mortality and longevity. These include (in part):

1. Gender: Mortality rates for females are lower at each age than those of men.
2. Genetics: There appears to be a link between genetic factors and mortality rates. Genetics may play a role in nine of the top-ten causes of death, according to the Centers for Disease Control and Prevention. The CDC lists the leading causes of death in the United States as cancer, chronic lower respiratory disease, accidents, stroke or cerebrovascular disease, Alzheimer's disease, diabetes, influenzas and pneumonia, kidney disease, and suicide.
3. Prenatal and childhood conditions: Poor conditions in utero, at birth, and in very early childhood are associated with mortality even at advanced ages.
4. Education: Higher education levels are linked to higher socioeconomic status, and both are linked to improved longevity, according to Hall and Peterson.
5. Socioeconomic status: As socioeconomic status decreases, so does life.

---

[197] Id.
[198] Id.
[199] Id.

6. Marital status: Married people have lower mortality rates than those who were never married, divorced, or widowed.

7. Ethnicity/migrant status: According to 2011 data compiled by the CDC, life expectancy is highest among Hispanic people, both male and female.

8. Lifestyle: See "Free Antiaging Life Extension Available to All."

9. Medical technology: The development of antibiotics and immunizations, as well as improvements in imaging, surgery, cardiac care, and organ transplants, all have helped push the average life expectancy higher.[200]

---

[200] K. Beckman, "9 Factors That Affect Longevity," https://www.thinkadvisor.com/2016/05/27/9-factors-that-affext-longevity.

6

survey on Acceptance of Extended Life

The Pew Research Center's Religion and Public Life Project conducted a survey of Americans seeking to determine their attitudes regarding radical life extension. Following is a summary of their findings. As you review the data, determine your response to each category and record your opinions within the appropriate area. Do your opinions fall within the majority of Americans, or are you in the minority? Some of the Pew survey findings are surprising.

Respondents to the following surveys provided their opinions without any insights being provided about radical life extension or regarding their health or youth status as the years increased. Whatever perceptions were held by the respondents as they considered their answers were not influenced by those who conducted the survey beforehand.

Views About Aging: To What Age Would You Like to Live?
Percent saying they want to live to age ...

78 or less	79-100	101-120	121 or more	Do not know	Median age
U.S Adults	14	69	4	4	9 = 100	90[201]

---

[201] Pew Research Center Survey Views, "About Aging. To What Age Would You Like To Live?" March 21–April 8, 2013.

Surprisingly, 69 percent of respondents elected a maximum life extension of between seventy-nine and one hundred years, while 14 percent did not desire a life expectancy beyond seventy-eight years. The desire to live beyond one hundred years drops dramatically to only 4 percent. The median life span is ninety years.[202]

Those individuals who would elect to live beyond one hundred years would typically desire to live as long as life-extending treatments could take them. These extended lifers would also not believe that their prolonged life is detrimental to society, at least not to the extent that they would forgo their efforts to live as long as possible.

Personal Desire for Life Extension, By Preferred Life Span
Percent saying they personally would or would not want medical treatments to extend life.

Would want	Would not want	Do not know
Ideal lifespan no more than 100	36 59 5	
Ideal lifespan 101 or more	67 29 4	

Within the above category, the influencing factor involves the administration of medical treatments in order to extend life. The larger number of respondents at 59 percent did not desire to have medical treatments to extend their lives beyond one hundred years. This would more likely be based upon a current assumption that life-extending medical treatments would involve artificial methods to maintain life, which many consider a life not worth living any longer, especially since the perception of such seniors would involve a frail and decrepit existence.

However, when the life span exceeds one hundred years, there is a converse opinion at 67 percent where now there is a dramatic increase in respondents desiring appropriate medical treatments to extend

---

[202] Id.

their lives. It appears that an extended life over one hundred years does not include the trepidation of a decrepit existence as envisioned for seniors who could live up to one hundred years.

A life existence over one hundred years crosses a threshold where there is greater confidence in medical science that focuses on medical treatments directed solely at extending life and not just maintaining life.

Views on Radical Life Extension, By Preferred Life Span
Percent saying medical treatments to extend life by decades would be a good or bad thing for society.

	Good for society	Bad for society	Do not know
Ideal lifespan no more than 100	41	54	5
Ideal lifespan 101 or more[203]	62	32	6

There are some similarities in this category as compared to the preceding category, although the focus here is with society, whereas the preceding category pertains to the individual. Here again, the perception of a life span no more than one hundred years is largely considered as bad for society. These respondent opinions evidently believe that the elder population in this category place an unreasonable burden upon society, the government, and others to support these ever-expanding elderly numbers.

Yet again there is another transition from a 54 percent majority who consider a life span of no more than one hundred years to be bad for society to a majority of 62 percent who consider a life span over 101 years as good for society. Evidently respondents believe the financial burdens and other problems associated with the care of the

---

[203] Pew Research Center Survey, "Radical Life Extension," https://www.pewforum. org/2013/08/06/chapter-3-views-about-aging/decades.

elderly in the under one hundred-year group are not represented with the life span of the 101-or-more group.

How Views Toward the Aging Population Relate to Views on Radical Life Extension

Having More Elderly People in the Population
Percent saying this trend is a good thing, a bad thing, or doesn't make much difference for American society

	Good thing	Doesn't make difference	Bad thing
U.S. adults	41	47	10[204]

Surprisingly, only 10 percent of respondents believed that having more elderly people in the population was a bad thing. Society in general is receptive to a senior population irrespective of the obvious financial burdens typically associated with the care of a senior population (e.g., Social Security, Medicare and other governmental health care programs, social services, long-term care, etc.).

After retirement, seniors typically transition from contributing to the economy to taking from the economy in areas described previously. Nonetheless, the government continues to place a high priority on providing financial support and services for the elderly population, especially with an ever-increasing senior population that brings significant political recognition with it.

With the equation shifting from a positive benefit to a negative draw for retired seniors, society remains vastly in favor of supporting an elderly population. However, the above category also indicates an acceptance of an elderly population during their normal life span without life-extension treatments beyond what is typically administered during routine medical care for seniors.

---

[204] Pew Research Center Survey Id., "Having More Elderly People in the Population," https://www.pewforum.org/2013/08/06/chapter-3-views-about-aging/decades.

Views on Radical Life Extension By Views on Having More Elderly in Population
Percent saying medical treatments to extend life by decades would be a good or bad thing for society.

Larger elderly population	Good for society	Bad for society	Do not know
Is a good thing	45	46	8
Makes no difference	42	52	6
Is a bad thing	26	71	3[205]

The notable difference in this category, when compared with the preceding category involving an elderly population, focuses upon including medical treatments to further extend life, whereas the above category does not.

The change in respondent opinions appears to indicate that when medical treatments are required to maintain or extend life, such efforts reflect a negative benefit to society, especially as pertains to the financial burdens placed upon society to care for an expanding elder population.

Population Growth and Life Extension World Population Growth and Resource Strains
Percent saying the growing world population will or will not be a major problem.

	Will not be a major problem	Will be a major problem
U.S. adults	37	61[206]

The majority of respondents (61 percent) indicate a pessimistic view in the world's ability to resolve an overpopulation problem

[205] Id.
[206] Pew Research Center Survey, "World Population Growth and Resource Strains," https://www.pewforum.org/2013/08/06/chapter-3-views-about-aging/decades.

resulting from a life-extension program as relating to available resources required to sustain itself. These respondents believe that an overpopulated society, including a majority of seniors, cannot be provided with adequate food, health care, and other necessary resources to sustain itself.

However, it would be more likely that a foreseeable overpopulation problem would not be caused by the number of individuals whose lives are extended by applicable medical intervention, per se, but rather due to the general health-care provisions implemented over time, resulting in longer life. Moreover, the increase in population would be negligible when considering those individuals who participated in a radical life-extension program because this group would be limited to the very few who could afford the high cost for the medical treatment.

Resolution of anticipated future overpopulation problems must be resolved by governmental agencies and other think tanks who address this critical issue and implement appropriate corrective measures well in advance, which, in my opinion, has not and most likely will not occur.

The change in respondent opinions appears to indicate that when medical treatments are required to maintain or extend life, such efforts reflect a negative benefit to society, especially as pertains to the financial burdens placed upon society to care for an expanding elder population.

These overpopulation problem-solvers must function, for the most part, independent of efforts to advance the benefits of medical research. In order to maintain the continued unabated advances in medical science that avail new innovations to benefit humanity, any potential inhibiting factors that could slow the forward progress of medical research must be identified and resolved in advance before progress is intimidated. Other potential inhibiting factors to forward progress could involve ethical concerns, religious beliefs, government intervention, FDA regulations, and law.

Views on Radical Life Extension, By Views on World Population Growth

Percent saying medical treatments to extend life by decades would be a good or bad thing for society

	Good thing	Bad thing	Do not know
World population growth			
Will be a major problem	33	61	6
Will not be a major problem	56	37	7[207]

The majority of respondents (61 percent) again believe the use of medical treatments to extend life, especially by decades, would be a bad thing. They believe that advancements in medical treatments may further complicate the overpopulation problem because such treatments will further increase the population numbers with more people living longer.

Personal Desire for Life Extension, By Views on World Population Growth

Percent saying they personally would or would not want medical treatments to extend life by decades

	Would want	Would not want	Do not know
World population growth will be a major problem.	34	61	5
Will not be a major problem	44	48	8[208]

---

[207] Pew Research Center Survey, "World Population Growth," https://www. pewforum.org/2013/08/06/chapter-3-views-about-aging/decades.

[208] Pew Research Center Survey, "Personal Desire for Life Extension," https:// www. pewforum.org/2013/08/06/chapter-3-views-about-aging/decades.

In this category, respondents (61 percent) who believe that overpopulation would be a problem for society also would reject medical treatments to obtain radical life extension. Similarly, those who say population growth will be a major problem for society are also less inclined to say they personally would want life-extending treatments. 34 percent would want treatment, compared with 44 percent among those who think world population growth will not be a major problem for society.[209]

Who Wants to Live Decades Longer?

Percent of U.S. adults saying (they personally/most people) would or would not want medical treatments that slow the aging process and allow the average person to live decades longer, to at least 120 years

	Would not want	Would want
They, personally	56	38
Most people	27	68[210]

---

[209] Pew Research Center Survey, "Living to 120 and Beyond: Americans. Views on Aging, Medical Advances and Radical Life Extension," https://www.pewforum.org/2013/08/06/living-to-120-and-beyond-americans-views-on-aging-medical-advances-and-radical-life-extension.

[210] Pew Research Center Survey, "Who Wants to Live Decades Longer?"

7

What Effects Would Overpopulation Have Upon Human Life Extension?

John Harris, a bioethicist at the University of Manchester, England, believes that the Earth can support only so many people. If everyone lived longer, generations would have to be born farther apart to avoid overcrowding.[211] Such attempts to monitor and regulate birth rates worldwide would be extremely difficult and most likely prove to be ineffective, while certain overall results would most likely prove to be inadequate.

Harris also postulates that to ensure ample generational turnover, society might need to resort to some kind of generational cleansing, which would be difficult to justify. This would involve people collectively deciding what length of life is reasonable for a generation to live and then ensuring individuals died once they reached the end of their term.[212]

The above horrifying future as envisioned by Harris was effectively depicted in the 1973 sci-fi drama *Soylent Green*, starring Charlton Heston and Edward G. Robinson. The film depicts that

---

[211] K. Than, "The Ethical Dilemmas of Immortality," https://www.livescience.com/10465-ethical-dilemmas-immortality.html.
[212] Id.

in the year 2022, New York City has exploded to a population of 40 million, where citizens must suffer the consequences of both severe overpopulation and the dramatic effects of climate change where the temperature is never below 90 degrees and the atmosphere is poisoned. All-natural resources have been exhausted, and everything is scarce, especially water and food. Only the very rich have access to adequate living space, food, and basic comforts like taking a shower.

With the inability of the Earth's resources to provide adequate food to the overwhelming population, the country's decision-makers have surreptitiously resorted to producing an artificial nutritious product supposedly made from plankton taken from the oceans. Later in the film, it is discovered that the actual ingredients of the cookie-like product, heretofore unknown to the public, are actually made from dead bodies.

Societies ultimately addresses the overpopulation problem by providing a gigantic euthanasia center known as "Home," where individuals who have had enough of living such a deprived and hopeless existence can freely elect to visit Home and be euthanized. There is also an apparent requirement that when people reach a certain age, they are required to go Home. Similar themes are played out in other sci-fi movies.

It is interesting to note that *Soylent Green* envisioned such a dysfunctional and horrifying consequences occurring in the year 2022, the concluding year of this writing. Fleischer may have based the target date for his described cataclysmic event to conclude in the year 2022 based upon his 1973 assessment of future trends involving overpopulation and environmental hazards to occur in 2022.

While certain aspects of this dramatic movie correlate with Harris' view that an overpopulated society may be obligated to limit the period of an individual's life span to a predetermined number of years, it certainly would not be expected that converting human corpses into a form of Soylent Green, in essence resorting to cannibalism, would ever occur. Although one could speculate that under certain conditions, such drastic consequences of a starving population would and indeed have occurred. Fleischer's drama presents the speculative effects of a society where both the tragedy of overpopulation and the dramatic failure of a polluted environment have combined to cause the ultimate terminating consequence for humanity.

As we consider the ever-advancing and unabated threats to our humanity based on a continually and dramatically-increasing population occurring in sync with the destruction of our environment, there is the proverbial line in the sand where, upon once crossed, there is no safe, effective, or corrective return. For example, consider the ever-expanding population of our world and the tragic consequences associated with the eventual reality that the world can no longer support the essential life requirements to sustain itself.

As of April 25, 2021, the world's population was estimated to be 7.867 billion. The population is expected to reach between 8 and 10.5 billion between 2040 and 2050. In 2017, the United Nations increased the medium variant projection to 9.8 billion for 2050 and 11.2 billion for 2100.[213] Now, consider the following historic list of the world's population growth:

Year	Billions	Years Between
1804	1	
1927	2	
1959	3	
1974	4	
1987	5	
1999	6	
2011	7	
2021	7.8[214]	

Therefore, since it has been predicted that the number of humans that Earth can sustain long term is about 1.9 billion people, roughly the global population about one hundred years ago in 1919, it can be

[213] "Human Overpopulation," en.wikipedia.org/wiki/Human Over population.
[214] Id.

surmised that the world's population has been extracting resources from the Earth at levels that cannot be adequately replaced since that time.

Rich Western countries are now siphoning up the planet's resources and destroying its ecosystem at an unprecedented rate. We have triggered a major extinction event. A world population of around a billion would have an overall pro-life effect. This could be supported for many millennia and sustain many more human lives in the long term compared with our current uncontrolled growth and prospects of a sudden collapse. If everyone consumed resources at the U.S. level, which is what the world aspires to, you will need another four or five Earths. We are wrecking our planet's life support system.[215]

The ultimate deciding factor, relevant to such issues, should typically be determined based on the simple risk-to-benefit analysis. If this process is applied, then forward progress and achievements in medicine, science, and other areas that are beneficial to humanity would usually prove to be of greater benefit than the perceived risks and negative aspects voiced by those who condemn and oppose a potential greater good. The concerns about overpopulation resulting from extending life beyond the standard life cycle is voiced by many as a major factor in opposing such efforts.

Overpopulation is certainly a valid and justifiable concern, both now and especially for the foreseeable future. The Earth retains limited resources in almost every category required to maintain and sustain life, and its capability to provide for all humanity will continue to be challenged as we scrape the bottom of the bucket.

If permanent and viable alternatives to support an ever-expanding population are not implemented immediately (most likely too late), it would be difficult to support scientific efforts that ultimately extend life, especially when and if radical life-extension treatments become available to a larger population beyond just the rich and powerful.

It is predicted that as life expectancy increases, the world population is aging at much higher rates. In fact, the number of

---

[215] Id.

people aged sixty and above is increasing at a rate of approximately 3 percent per year.[216] Currently, there are 962 million people aged sixty and above across the globe, according to the most recent estimates. By the year 2050, this number is projected to more than double, and the number of people aged eighty and above is expected to triple.[217]

However, I do not believe that overpopulation will become a legitimate argument to deter continued scientific exploration to discover answers to humanity's worthy pursuit for continued youth, defeating the aging process, and extending life and awareness.

This opinion is also based upon another ageless reality. Those who have wealth and power will be the very few who could afford the anticipated high cost of reducing the continue encroachment of the inevitable aging process and thus will be the select participants to extend their lives.

Moreover, it is highly doubtful that medical insurance companies in the future will pay the exorbitant cost for radical life-extension treatments, thereby effectively preventing the average American from receiving life-extending treatments. They will simply argue that such large expenditures are not appropriate because the treatment falls outside the normal and natural range of typical life expectancy, in a manner akin to elective surgery. Furthermore, if medical insurance companies were required to pay for radical life-extension treatments, which would open the door to a much larger patient population, the cost of medical insurance for all would increase dramatically.

It is amazing to me when considering the enormous overindulging societies of the world, especially as it pertains to the more prosperous countries like the United States and the vastly overpopulated extent of our world that society has dramatically failed long ago to respond in an appropriate manner to the blatantly obvious reality that our daily consumption of essential life products cannot nearly be replaced. The math is simple and unambiguous. We are using up our vital resources

---

[216] Id.
[217] Id.

necessary to sustain our existence much faster than the world has the capability to replace.

We have been existing on borrowed time and resources with no apparent viable intent to correct the inevitable catastrophic calamity that awaits us just over the hill. Unless the world's governments can unite in a consolidated effort to effectively resolve the hazards involving overpopulation and relatively soon, population growth will continue unabated with related famine, disease, pestilence, and wars. Here again, this issue, as critical as it is to the continued existence of humanity, is a separate and independent concern and therefore must be addressed as such. It is not a choice of one or the other.

Concluding Opinion

As you can also conclude by extrapolating the summary data and details provided previously and in other publications, it is clearly evident that we have already crossed the line of no return with little potential ability to resolve the inevitable calamity to our society that may conclude in a world that can no longer nourish its people and subsequently exacts a great toll in the suffering and death of great numbers.

Prediction

Any reasonable conclusion, after reviewing facts available to anyone who cares enough to look, will more likely than not conclude that it is inevitable that our society will eventually experience a critical shortage of resources that have hitherto been available with little or no concern about the world's ability to continue supplying such demands and expectations.

We have witnessed, even here in the United States, how a population will react when they believe there may be a shortage of a vital resource. For example, when the COVID-19 virus initially became apparent, there was an immediate and overwhelming surge by a fearful population that decimated the shelves of grocery stores. Or when there appeared to be a pending shortage of gasoline, the lines at gas stations stretched for blocks.

Whenever the tipping point arrives, most likely within the foreseeable future, it will happen with an immediate worldwide panic that will strip every source of food, water, fuel, and other life-supporting necessities available throughout the world. Society at large will disintegrate into a realm involving a tumultuous, out-of-control uprising with great fear and threatening mobs roaming the land, seeking to obtain vital goods by whatever means necessary. And yet, even with the reality that such a horrendous and unfathomable catastrophic event of biblical proportions may be just beyond the horizon, there has been little appropriate recognition that any corrective measures need be taken.

I have hesitated to provide you with my ultimate prediction on this issue because of the fear and trepidation it may cause you; however, based upon the intent behind my putting this book together, I will offer the following. Please remember that my opinions, predictions, and the following portray only my conclusions, while many other notable authorities in related fields of study would disagree with my final assessment.

Nonetheless, it is my concluding opinion on the subject of overpopulation that it is already too late to stop the inevitable reality to the approach of worldwide starvation and the dramatic effects that will befall humanity based upon the data and information indicated previously and through other documented scientific evidence to support such a conclusion.

The warning signs have been staring worldwide humanity in the face for many decades while humankind has continued to overindulge from the limitations of the world's resources without appropriate recognition and response to adequately and appropriately replenish what has been harvested.

The ability of the world to further supply the gluttonous appetite for essential resources required to sustain an exploding population is simply not tenable and will eventually, within the foreseeable future, just collapse with unfathomable and truly devastating consequences. The ignorance or oblivious, uninhibited, self-indulgence of our limited resources (e.g., food, water, forests, oceans, air quality, etc.) will just collapse with only a limited ability to provide too little to so many.

While there is a large population of individuals referred to as survivalists, many of whom have invested significant amounts of money and effort in preparing for such a cataclysmic eventuality or other catastrophic event, with underground facilities and large quantities of provisions, even these long-term survival expectations are limited to only a few years.

History has provided recorded evidence in many countries that illustrates how a society will react when it is deprived of necessary items they deem to be required for their continued existence. Countries have gone to war to forcefully acquire necessary materials and provisions they can no longer provide for themselves. Often countries, especially the United States, have interceded by providing aid to such countries in need; however, if the entire world suffers from such catastrophic events, there will be no opportunity for the world to resurrect itself to the blissful abundance of resources it once had available.

So why so much emphasis on overpopulation? In my estimation, progression toward overpopulation is antagonist and distracting to purposes that support life-extension research and similar endeavors. For example, as the awareness of the ever-evolving hazards of overpopulation becomes more apparent to governments, other vested groups, and participating scientists, the resistance to support activities to extend life will become more recognized and profound with the passage of time. The continued emphasis and drive to extend life will be perceived as counterproductive and non sequitur to the reality of an ever-expanding population that lacks the ability to support its further existence as a whole.

Therefore, funding could begin to dwindle, and the once-enthusiastic support for the invested scientists, government, and society in general could gradually evaporate. Any successful accomplishment in the fields of scientific research focused upon extending life might not receive the warranted accolades of such historic and anticipated scientific accomplishments. Quite to the contrary, any recognized accomplishments within any medical or scientific endeavor that contributes to the further extension of human life may be viewed as heading in the wrong direction.

There was a time when mothers who propagated many children were recognized as heroes in supporting the advancement of civilization and humanity. However, as it became apparent that the population of the world's communities was increasing to problematic levels, the opposite opinions were expressed to those mothers who had large numbers of children. Some countries, like China, went as far as to impose limits on the number of children that a family could have.

However, regardless of the effects that an overpopulated society may have upon scientific medical research to extend life, I do not believe that the focused emphasis and enthusiastic scientific endeavors to extend the longevity of human life would be thwarted. While much of the more dramatic methods of extending life, such as brain and head transplants, are speculated for far future possibilities, other areas of life-extending technologies may be available in the foreseeable or near future, including the combination of AI humanoid robots and transferred, uploaded human memories, including awareness and conscience.

In other words, I anticipate that near-future, technological accomplishments that would actually extend human life will occur and not be inhibited by the problems associated with an overpopulated society. There will always be the wealthy and powerful to influence such endeavors that they perceive to be of particular significance and value to their own self-interest as the concept of extending their lives would undoubtedly provide a compelling motivation for them to assure that such life-extending innovations will indeed be accomplished.

One final thought on this subject of overpopulation: The ultimate salvation of our continued existence may not be dependent upon any corrective measures initiated by humanity, which has failed in a continual and dismal manner to alleviate or inhibit the inevitable movement toward self-extinction. History has clearly demonstrated that nations would more easily go to war rather than consolidate their available resources and capabilities toward protecting our environment and its ability to provide the necessary essentials required to maintain our continued existence.

Therefore, in the future when artificial intelligence (AI) becomes a reality, assuming our existence will continue until then, the uninhibited mental processing of artificial thought, free from the external influence of political self-interest groups, the wealthy, the military, and other worldwide decision-makers that have and will continue to permit the catastrophic demise of our existence, the clarity of appropriate decisions may finally initiate the necessary corrective measures that may save our planet and our existence. However, as I predicted earlier, the ability of our planet to continue providing the necessary resources to sustain the population would most likely have already failed, in other words, too little too late.

Depending upon how advanced the AI entities would have evolved and the relationship between the AI and humans, these artificial thinkers would not depend on any of the resources so critical to humanity. The implications of such a possibility, including continued awareness, is discussed later in this book.

8

Petri Dish Existence

Perhaps the earliest attempts at postponing the inevitable demise of our awareness at the moment our physical body is near death or immediately after death would be the removal of the human brain from the head and to maintain its capacity to exist without the body. If this could be accomplished within the foreseeable future, distant future, or ever, the objective would be to sustain and maintain as much, if not all, of the cognitive awareness that existed within the brain before the physical death of the body that hitherto maintained the existence of the brain and awareness.

The physical status of the brain during its removal and subsequent isolated and maintained existence after removal would be the highest priority. Currently, no surgical procedure or technology would enable a successful process to remove a human brain and sustain its existence. The surgical procedure would be extremely difficult, time-consuming, and arduous. However, three renowned neuroscientists believe it is possible to remove a human brain from a body and place it in a tank at an interim holding facility where living brains could hypothetically be stored, waiting transplantation.[218]

---

[218] N. Ungerleider, "Not Science Fiction: A Brain In A Box to Let People Live on After Death, https://www.fastcompany.com/3015553/not-science-fiction-a-brain-in-a-box-to-let-people-live-on-after-death.

Even if there should come a time in the future when neuroscientists and others devised a procedure to remove the brain and maintain its cognitive existence, there would remain a high probability that the brain would fail to maintain its vital status and ultimately die before the process would be completed. This conclusion would be particularly significant if the attempt involved the separation of the brain from its spinal cord.

Moreover, there would be no method to effectively determine how successful such a post-surgical procedure concluded since there would be no method of having the brain communicate its post-procedural status to the scientists, other than very basic telemetry feedback, such as placing electrodes on the surface of the isolated brain to detect electrical signals indicating brain activity, although to a limited extent.

Now, consider the potential existence of an awakened brain with its cognitive ability to comprehend its existence after its brain is removed and retained in a state of perpetual artificial existence. Try to imagine that you retain an awareness of your existence and prior memories, thoughts, feelings, and emotions in a black void without the ability to experience any of your basic senses. You cannot hear, see, feel, taste, or experience any form of cognitive existence other than being aware that you can think and recall prior memories.

Moreover, you have no ability to communicate your desires or any form of information to those who reside in a different reality. You could not even terminate your own existence if you chose to do so. While the sustained brain remains in a suspended realm of continued, unabated, and inhibited awareness, there would be no apparent ability to turn off the thinking process until it was time for the implantation or until the brain fails. Thus, the awakened brain would exist in a continual realm of waiting. It is not known whether you could dream or sense the passage of time. You would most likely not experience sleep and would ponder your experience continually.

So why would any individual possibly consider availing themselves to such a horrible and terrifying experience? The most likely answer is because the transplanted brain offers, regardless how remote the possibility, that their existence and awareness could continue after their normal life cycle existence was forced to terminate, or

117

near termination, because the body could no longer sustain itself. Many individuals, especially those who dramatically fear death, would accept any potential possibility that provides them with an opportunity to continue their experience of life, even if such life involves an artificial means of their continued awareness.

The primary objective would be to preserve their awareness and other key cognitive abilities in the isolated brain for as long as possible with the hope that the brain would retain its awareness capacity until such time as technology would enable a brain transplant to another body or upload the brain's memories and stored information from the brain into a computer or other mechanism capable of receiving, storing, and retrieving the stored information.

One significant, unknown concern pertains to the quality of the brain's retained awareness and stored information. If indeed the thinking brain were waiting for the time of its transplantation or possibility for its awareness transfer, would the cognitive processing ability at the eventual time of implantation retain the same level of acuity as it had when removed and placed within the holding facility? Would it be possible for continued awareness in a dark, blank realm, for any amount of time or even more so for an expanded period of time, to not suffer some level of degraded awareness or consciousness? There could be no ability to determine if the cognitive processes of the transplanted brain maintained sufficient and adequate effective comprehension to warrant the transplant or transferred procedure.

Based upon research and experiments conducted by Yale University neuroscientist Nenad Sestan and his research team involving pig brains, he was able to conclude that it is conceivable that the brain could be kept alive indefinitely and that steps could be attempted to restore awareness. However, his team elected not to do either because "this is uncharted territory."[219]

---

[219] A. Regalado, "Researchers are keeping pig brains alive outside the body," https://www.technologyreview.co/2018/04/25/240742/researchers-are-keeping-pig-brains-alive-outside-the-body.

In my opinion, Sestan's conclusion is pointless because most scientific research will venture into uncharted territory. That's why it's referred to as research. Moreover, why would Sestan and his team terminate their study after it appears they were at a pinnacle point of scientific discovery that beckoned further and continued pursuit for greater insights and understanding? Sestan's justification for terminating his study is difficult to understand and reconcile.

An isolated brain is a brain kept alive *in vitro* (an artificial environment outside the living body),[220] either by perfusion, a blood substitute, often an oxygenated solution of various salts, or submersion of the brain in oxygenated artificial cerebrospinal fluid.[221]

With the brain being considered a living organ before the transfer, the definition of something living would no longer be applicable once the information is received by the computer or any other artificial receiving technology. Thus, a dramatic transition from a living organism to a non-living entity would have occurred.

There is, however, an apparent insurmountable dilemma that presents itself to the sponsor, neuroscientific team, medical surgeons, FDA, law, and especially any potential candidates for the subject procedure or similar procedures. I cannot conceive how any sponsor who intends to remove the human brain and maintain its vitality in vitro or any other method of viable suspension could possibly receive approval from the FDA or any appropriate legal authority to do so. There is simply no route through the stringent clinical study regulations and applicable laws that would permit human trials in order to effectively respond to prerequisite requirements for safety, effectiveness, and reliability, at least not for the foreseeable future. Such an endeavor would require a totally new and unique pathway for all participants involving new regulations, laws, and prerequisite accomplishments to be established and implemented. Neuroscientists and bioethicists, including Dr. Sestan, published

---

[220] "In vitro," The American Heritage Dictionary, Second College Edition.
[221] "Isolated Brain," en.wikipedia.org/wiki/Isolated Brain.

an editorial arguing that experiments on human brain tissue may require special protections and rules.[222]

I am absolutely convinced that very restrictive new laws, regulations, guidelines, and any other involved participant concerns would be required well in advance of approving any such surgical procedures and involve countless review meetings before a reasonable and consolidated consensus could be achieved. Moreover, specific regulations and law also speak to the rights, safety, and welfare of the human subjects potentially involved in the investigation.[223]

Today, as I attempt to conceive how the government and lawmakers could possibly accomplish the development of required new regulations and laws for the neurological applications discussed in this book, especially for near-future neurological procedures. I cannot imagine how such an endeavor could be achieved in a legal or regulatory-compliant manner.

Conceivably, it may prove more difficult to maneuver through the non-tangible aspects of neurological research and discovery involving the entanglements of new regulations, laws, ethics, and other inhibiting factors than the actual efforts of neuroscientists and other participants to perform their scientific investigations and research activities.

Another approach was proposed by Robert McIntyre, MIT graduate and co-founder of Nectome. McIntyre's new venture intends to preserve the brain of people, like the thirty individuals who have paid $10,000 to have his company preserve their brains for future uploading. McIntyre has stated that what we're focused on is preserving long-term memory that currently does not exist.[224]

Countering McIntyre's perspective, McGill University neuroscientist Michael Hendricks believes that McIntyre's claims

---

[222] A. Regalado, "Researchers are keeping pig brains alive outside the body."

[223] Code of Federal Regulations (CFR). Food and Drugs. Parts 800-1299. Revised April 1, 2017. Investigational Device Exemptions (IDE). Subparts 812.25, 812.27, 812.30, and 812.35.

[224] S. Begley, "After ghoulish allegations, a brain-preservation company seeks redemption," https://www.statnews.com/2019/01/30/nectome-brain-preservation-redemption.

offer abjectly false hope by transhumanists promising resurrection in ways that technology can probably never deliver.[225]

For Nectome's procedure to work, it is essential that the brain be fresh. The company says "its plan is to connect people with terminal illnesses to a heart-lung machine in order to pump its mix of scientific embalming chemicals into the big carotid arteries in their neck while they are still alive, although under general anesthesia." The procedure is 100 percent fatal.[226]

Edward Boyden, an MIT neuroscientist, has stated his concern that future participants are fully informed of what we do know and what we don't know about the process.[227] The unknowns, of course, are substantial. Not only does no one know what consciousness is, it will be hard to tell if an eventual simulation has any, says Boyden.[228]

---

[225] A. Regalado, "A startup is pitching a mind-uploading service that is '100 percent fatal'," https://www.technologyreview.com/2018/03/13/144721/a-startup-is-pitching-a-mind-uploading-service-that-is-100-percent-fatal.
[226] Id.
[227] Id.
[228] S. Begley, "After ghoulish allegations, a brain-preservation company seeks redemption."

9

Ethical Considerations Involving Longevity Research

It would not be fair to say the research scientists involved in pushing the outer limits of the aging process do not consider the ethical implications of their efforts and discoveries. However, I believe it would also be fair to say that ethical consideration will ultimately not hamper scientific endeavors to accomplish their objective goals of extending life as far as possible.

If the research efforts of these scientists were constantly scrutinized by various ethical overseers, individuals, and groups and constantly challenged by the focus of their inquiry, then research itself would be inhibited, distracted, and disrupted. Moreover, ethical considerations are as varied and subjective as the individual who puts forth their opinion on the subject. Nonetheless, this is not to suggest that ethical influence and monitoring are absent from the field of research involving the brain, head transplants, awareness transfers, AI humanoid robots, and so forth.

Neuroethics, a sub-field of bioethics that has emerged in the past fifteen years, intends to ensure that technologies that directly affect the brain are developed in an ethical manner.[229] Neuroethicist

---

[229] L. Drew, "The ethics of brain-computer interfaces," https://www.nature.com/articles/d41586-019-02214-2.

Marcello Ienca at the Swiss Federal Institute of Technology in Zurich, has stated,

> We don't want to be the watchdog of neuroscience or to police how neurotechnology should be developed. Instead, those in the field want to see ethics integrated into the initial design and development stages of such technologies, to maximize their benefits and to identify and minimize their potential harm—whether to individuals or to a wider society[230] before their intended use is approved and released for commercial use.

The review and approval process of any new technology by the FDA is not subjective and thus totally dependent upon scientific data and details and not on intangible opinions or conclusions based solely on ethical considerations to approve or disapprove controversial research projects.

However, it is quite evident with the progressive advent of neurological research involving brain preservation, brain transplants, mind uploading, and other life longevity research that an initial ethical research approval process (based solely on the ethical implications of such research and especially anticipated clinical studies) should first be reviewed by an ethical review board.

The formality of such an ethical review board would also eliminate the potential for knee-jerk reactions during research or clinical studies between ethical oversight and research scientists, which could prove to be extremely frustrating and inhibiting to the further advancement of new medical technology, discovery, and development. The focus and expertise of these two entities, ethics and science, involve very different mindsets and may not constitute a happy, but hopefully, productive relationship.

We are currently living in a time when critical new issues never conceived of before now require that new laws, regulations, social

---

[230] Id.

conscience, religious convictions, and other influencing factors must be amalgamated into determining what is best for the individual, society, and humankind involving such expected radical surgical procedures. Conceivably, some of these non-tangible considerations may become prerequisite requirements that must be addressed before any neurological clinical studies or subsequent procedure can commence.

The ethical implications and biases associated with scientific efforts to extend human life are more profound now than ever before. There are two rigid opinion camps, each as adamant and steadfast as the other in their views on this subject.

Pijnenburg and Leget argue that research with the explicit aim of extending the human life span is both undesirable and morally unacceptable. They present three serious objections relating to justice, the community, and the meaning of life. These authors hold the opinion, "We think that there is a fundamental difference between the desirability of being alive within the limits of the average life expectancy and the desirability of being alive beyond those limits."[231] They summarize their argument against extending the human life span as follows (brief excerpts):

Justice

The most obvious moral problem is the already existing unequal death.[232] In other words, their premise is based upon an observation that those individuals who would benefit from life-extending treatments will only be the rich and powerful (e.g., "the way of the world").

While the ethical implication recognizes the reality and disparity between the poor and the lower-class members of a society and the

---

[231] C. Pijnenburg et al., "Who wants to live forever? Three arguments against extending the human lifespan," *Journal of Medical Ethics* 33 (10): 585–587. Doi: 10.1136/jme. 2006-017822. https://www.ncbi.nih.gov/pmc/articles/ PMC2652797.
[232] Id.

wealthy and powerful class, it would not be ethically or morally prudent to deny access to life-extending treatments to only those who can afford these amenities. For example, if the same life-extending benefits could not be provided for everyone, regardless of their ability to afford such treatments, it could be argued that no one should receive the treatments to extend their life.

To the contrary, it would be unethical and immoral to deny extended life services to the wealthy based on the reality that others in the world cannot afford the same. Nothing is gained or recognized as a positive factor in denying additional years of life to the privileged few.

Of course, this reality would leave us with the frustration and unfairness of such a system; however, it would not constitute an injustice within the concept of justice (i.e., right or wrong), but rather within the eyes of humanity, it would be perceived as unjust, but nonetheless not unlawful or even unethical. The only apparent approach to resolving this dilemma would appear to rest within the government to implement controls, especially financial and procedure availability, for those who provide treatments targeted at extending life.

While the government's intervention may not completely level the playing field, it should avail the benefits of extended life opportunities to a greater portion of society and throughout the world, but obviously not everyone.

However, I am not optimistic that the government, especially that of the United States, would ever implement any regulations or influence upon those who are the givers of life-extension treatments because the cost to produce their treatments involving drugs or more advanced methods and technologies would prove to be financially prohibited in providing for such a large population.

Only if the government were motivated to subsidize these entities with significant amounts of funding would they be willing to avail their products and procedures to a larger segment of the population. Nonetheless, it would be difficult for the government to support such an effort unless the cost was dramatically reduced and other political, economic, and ethical issues were resolved.

Therefore, as life has provided a distinct advantage throughout the millenniums to the wealthy and powerful, it appears that those who will experience a chance for extended life will continue to be limited to only the rich and powerful and perhaps only a limited number of those.

Pijnenburg and Leget thus conclude, "Our efforts to prolong life, therefore, ought not to be separated from the more fundamental questions relating to integrity, given the problem of unequal death, can we morally afford to invest in research to extend life."[233]

While ethical and moral consideration should always weigh in on such relevant issues as maintaining and extending life, they should not restrain the forward progress of inquiry and research that would ultimately benefit humanity. To press forward is an innate desire of humanity to discover the unknown on the other side of the hill. This is especially true for those who pursue discovery and advancements in science and medicine. There are those who would, and have, argued the ethical and moral disadvantageous of research and discoveries that have prolonged life even as it pertains to early medical cures and treatments to the present.

With these individuals, there seems to be a perverse belief that nature or some other entity has established and ordained the status quo that where we are is where we ought to be. Consider where we would be or how we would have evolved if such ethical or moral restrictions had restrained our progress for a better, safer, healthier, and less troublesome life.

Community

Human beings are viewed as social beings: relations with others belong to the essentials of what it is to live a human life.[234] Living longer is valuable only if it results in living longer in meaningful relations. Quality of time outweighs quantity of time. The real ethical

---

[233] Id.
[234] Id.

challenge for aging societies, therefore, should be how to improve the conditions for life as a community and not how to stop aging as such.[235]

The authors place a greater emphasis: to improve the conditions for life as a community rather than attempt to address the aging problem. However, this is a separate and independent focus worthy of considerable effort but not related to the aging process. For example, individual communities would define different criteria for what would constitute for their community an acceptable or appropriate social environment, much of which might be governed by applicable laws, customs, and practices deemed appropriate for their lifestyle.

So let us assume that such a community was successful in establishing a harmonious environment within the confines of its citizens, which is doubtful. If there is one overriding reality that history has acknowledged and illustrated regarding community relationships, it is the fact that neighboring communities rarely get along. Eventually, one community, state, tribe, or government, regardless of how small or how big, will challenge the other in a dispute or even go to war with their neighbor.

Take, for example, the alliance of opposing countries during WWII, when China and Russia were our allies, while Germany and Japan were the enemies. Shortly after the war, these combative nations changed their allegiance where our allies became our enemies and our enemies became our allies. It makes absolutely no sense, but there it is.

For the authors' arguments of prioritizing meaningful relations with others, such unachievable objectives must encompass other communities outside the boundaries of any one community. Thus far, in the advancement of humankind and civilization, this worthy goal has seldom been accomplished.

If the requirements were to reach some undefined level of community relationship, harmony, and other prerequisite criteria, then efforts to address the aging problem would most likely never

---

[235] Id.

occur. Moreover, what does improving life within a community really mean? What is considered acceptable, and what is not? Trying to establish and implement a standard level of acceptance by a community does not provide sufficient emphasis on the relationship expectations of the individual. There are those who have no emotional problems being alone. Some will even prefer such independence, while others will desperately feel a need for relationships. Most of us are somewhere in between.

Pijnenburg and Leget argue that human beings cannot live without meaningful relations with others.[236] However, if this were true, then what would be the alternative? Moreover, how would one define a meaningful relationship? What would be the defined boundaries of an acceptable relationship or of some lacking relationship component? There are simply too many variables within the topic of community relationships to impose any limitations on efforts to establish a prescribed standard of acceptance by everyone. To devote efforts at resolving the aging problem is not only to focus on extending life beyond the accepted length of normal life expectancy, but also to reduce or eliminate pain and suffering that typically accompanies the elderly.

Pijnenburg and Leget focus their entire emphasis upon the benefits of community relationships while degrading any value or worthiness in pursuing efforts at resolving aging problems or prolonging life. They state that living longer is valuable only if it results in living longer in meaningful relations.[237] However, their entire argument prohibits any investment of time and effort to resolving problems associated with the aging process and extending life as if to do so would diminish the emphasis to focus on improving community relationships.

Moreover, upon what premise do these authors assume that their emphasis upon the quality of life versus the length of life would be limited only to those who live within their normal life expectancy?

---

[236] Id.

[237] Id.

Why would such emphasis of happiness and enhanced communal relationships not continue into the prolonged life?

The Meaning of Life

The authors third, and final, argument is,

> life extension as an explicit aim is contrary to the wisdom of ages as contained in various religious and non-religious spiritual traditions. Although all traditions agree that life is worthy, there is always a notion that human beings miss the essence of life by focusing on the preservation of their self or ego.[238]

Many spiritual and religious traditions make this point in the notion of truly human life by the decentring [e.g., remove or displace (the individual human subject, such as the author of a text) from a primary place or central role[239]] of the self.[240]

In summary, the author's arguments do not provide adequate justification for diminishing or disregarding scientific and medical advancements as targeted at resolving the aging problem or life extension. The arguments presented are far more appropriate for philosophical, religious, moral, and ethical discussions and debates.

The issues of moral and ethical dilemma as they relate to advancements within the medical scientific community have long presented their objections and opinions. While such implications are worthy of reflection, they should not present any serious restrictions or limitations regarding the forward progress of medical research directed at resolving the aging process or extended life.

---

[238] Id.

[239] "Decentring," https://www.google.com/search?q=decentring&riz=1CiOPRB_enUS580US590&oq=decentring&aqs=chrome..69i57j0j0i1013j0j0l04.17272j1j15&sour.

[240] C. Pijnenburg et al., "Who wants to live forever? Three arguments against extending the human lifespan."

Scientific endeavors to find answers and discoveries that ease the burden and suffering of the elderly and extend the length of life will not be diminished. The inquisitive mind cannot be stifled.

Also, the arguments posed by Pijnenburg and Leget appear not to be based on any empirical findings involving data or peer review literature that provides justifiable or validated support regarding their disapproval of efforts to focus on the aging problem or life extension. Their arguments are subjective at best.

Another author, Allen J. Frances, like many others, does not support attempts to address the problems associated with aging and life extension. Dr. Frances argues, "The world is already terribly over-populated and is rapidly becoming even more over-populated. Extending lifespan will mean more crowding, more mouths to feed, more environmental degradation, and more resource depletion."[241]

This provides some further support for my position on overpopulation discussed earlier. A longer life for some must be purchased at the high cost of a more brutal life for the many, a life threatened by even more wars, migrations, famines, and epidemics.[242]

While I agree with Dr. Frances' position on the serious problems associated with overpopulation, as discussed previously, here again is another anchor tied to the necks of research scientists who desire and have tailored their carriers to resolving the dilemma and mystery of the aging process and extended life.

Certainly, there have been, and always will be, continued adverse events such as described by Dr. Frances above. However, these should not diminish any emphasis on dealing with advances that reduce the suffering that typically accompanies aging. Thus, there exists a conflict between working at resolving the aging and overpopulation issues while also assuring scientific endeavors that continue to

---

[241] A. Frances, "A Debate on the Pros and Cons of Aging and Death," https://www.psychologytoday.com/us/blog/saving-normal/201612/debate-the-pros-and-cons-aging-and-death.

[242] C. Paddock, "Brain activity has role in human aging and longevity," https://www.medicalnewstoday.com/articles/#memory-loss324516.

address the aging problem and at extending life, both adding to the problem of overpopulation.

Most of the concerns identified above by Dr. Frances are not related to efforts at resolving the aging problem or life extension. These issues will require their own independent focus of investigation and analysis separate from any bearing on resolving aging issues.

To diminish or reduce the emphasis on research or any activity that attempts to extend the benefits to humanity is to deny the inherent destiny of humankind. The ingenuity and evolution in advancements of science, medicine, technology, and many other endeavors over a relatively short period of time is a testimony to the inquisitive nature of the human mind. Such forward-looking initiatives by humankind cannot and must not be diminished, inhibited, or unsupported by the government or any other opposing entities.

Dr. Frances also holds the opinion that there is no reason to believe it is scientifically feasible or ethically desirable for people to stay young for 150 years. The most compelling lesson of scientific research is that the body is far more complicated and intricately balanced than we could possibly imagine.[243] The abundance of scientific literature about longevity indicates significant progress in extending the length of human life.

While there are those scientists who support Dr. Frances' opinion, there are many who disagree and conclude that extended life has become and will continue to be a reality for both near and far future human existence.

This conclusion is particularly relevant as it pertains to the continued existence of awareness and memory as discussed throughout this reading, primarily because scientific research and discovery will place less dependence on the human body and more emphasis on artificial methods to extend the individual's life and awareness.

As greater progress and discovery become reality with the passage of time, less and less emphasis will be directed toward the more traditional methods to support human existence with greater

---

[243] A. Frances, "A Debate on the Pros and Cons of Aging and Death. Psychology Today."

emphasis being placed upon artificial treatments to extend life. These efforts will continue to capture the enthusiasm of medical researcher scientists to push harder with their research efforts.

While great advancements have been achieved in medicine and scientific research that now provide replacement components and organs throughout the human body, there is a current understanding that human life can be extended only so far. Current scientific thinking estimates the human body has a maximum extended life as stipulated by some scientists of 115,[244] 125,[245] and 150 to 200[246] years.

Dr. Frances' opinion that the body is far more complicated and intricately balanced than we could possibly imagine is the reality that all medical scientists and engineers have been burdened with to identify and resolve. And so, they have for centuries focused with greater clarity and understanding that continues to this day, and undoubtedly into the future, to find answers to the hidden secrets for healing and life extension within the human body.

The wonder and complexity of the human body is less a mystery with the passage of time and discovery. With continued advancements in resolving factors that inhibit a healthy and longer life, science will continue to reduce or even eliminate the unknown factors that restrain us from extending the life of humankind, although the outer limits remain speculative and contentious.

In Dr. Frances' initial opinion, he argues that there is no reason to believe it is scientifically feasible or ethically desirable for people to stay young for 150 years.[247] While the feasibility of living to 150 years or even much longer may not be feasible, as scientists on the negative side of longevity argue, I cannot discern any negative ethical implication associated with the ability to "stay young for 150 years," other than the overpopulation issue.

[244] "Aging," en.wikipedia.org/wiki.
[245] "Life extension," en.wikipedia.org.wiki/ Life extension.
[246] "Scientist thinks the world's first 200 year old person has already been born," https://norwaytoday.info/everyday/scientist-thinks-worlds-first-200-year-old person-already-born.
[247] A. Frances, "A Debate on the Pros and Cons of Aging and Death."

There are those who argue that extending life would be of little value if maintaining their youth failed to follow a parallel course with advancements in the aging process. I tend to agree with this assessment since simply to extend the life of an elder individual without the benefit of experiencing a somewhat youthful regeneration of that awareness would not offer a significant incentive to experience an extended life, at least not to many.

This is not to suggest that the middle-aged individual or even seniors should not have an equal opportunity to benefit from life-extension treatment. However, qualified candidates for medical intervention to extend their lives would most likely involve more stringent prerequisite criteria for older individuals than the younger candidates. This would be especially significant when such life-extending treatments initially become available.

Even if we assume that it were possible to retain one's youth to age 150, the subject is a moot point because the evolution and advances of the aging process and maintaining youth are two independent efforts. For example, two horses in a race will not run equally side by side for an extended time. One will eventually take the lead or fall behind. In this case, it appears that the pursuit of youth would most likely fall behind. Science will not be able to have both age-related pursuits and continued youth cross the finish line at the same time.

Although in the earlier phases of researching longevity and continued youth, there may be a parallel relationship; however, eventually extending life should win the race with advances in continued youth tagging behind. In other words, the enormous complexities of the human body and its multitude of idiosyncrasies required to function in a harmonious process to maintain life is a daunting task without the introduction of therapeutic prophylactic drugs and artificial devices at times when they are required to overcome inhibiting human health-related obstacles. Therefore, as advances in bioscientific discovery continue to extend human life, the dependency upon the body to maintain its existence will diminish with a greater dependency upon artificial processes to maintain and extend life.

There are those who reason that if they alone were to experience an extended life, their family members and friends would eventually die, and their cherished relationships would no longer be available to them. Of course, if other family members and friends were also willing to avail themselves to the extended life process and could afford the high cost of doing so, then those relationships would continue, although undoubtedly with fewer family members.

There is also another perspective to consider. If radical life extension were available and affordable to a larger population and if longevity were also accompanied with a youthful demeanor, then how would one reconcile a harmonious existence where their parents, grandparents, great-grandparents, and even great-great grandparents that exist within the same life-extending realm? How would each level of awareness relate to one another?

As noted throughout this discussion, as scientists continue to discover and implement advances in biomedicine, biotechnology, and other related scientific endeavors during their research pursuits, the acquisition of new knowledge will continue to remove the barriers that have hindered their forward progress. With each scientific advance, the length of life is extended further and further, facilitating yet greater discovery.

However, overpopulation would drain every social service funding program, including welfare, Social Security, Medicare, unemployment benefits, housing, and so forth. With the continued increase in population and the advancements in AI machines and robotic support technology, employment, especially for those with less education, will become a serious problem.

Those in Favor

Regardless of those who are opposed to the efforts focused on extending life, and there are many, there are those who support scientific endeavors to extend life as far as is scientifically possible. There are indeed two separate camps with little agreement between either.

From the time we enter elementary school through high school and perhaps college, we are formally engaged in the academic learning process followed by years of experience in our chosen career and life in general. It seems that when we are at the apex of our accumulated life experiences and knowledge, we start to fade with the advent of older age, resigning ourselves to retirement, even when it is imposed upon us by age limitation or other restrictions.

Following a life of hectic involvement with school, life, business, and the investments of our consolidated endeavors, we suddenly face a new and unexpected challenge when our busy daily schedule and demands suddenly give way to an awareness that we are no longer that productive individual that we once were. We seem to lose a sense of self-value and even dignity, sometimes feeling that the contributing aspects of our life are now gone.

After we initially enjoy certain aspects of our retirement, eventually we find ourselves sitting in a chair wondering, "What am I going to do now?" For some, depression will overtake their reality with the thoughts that their future destiny is awaiting their eventual demise.

Such is the reality of many Americans as they enter their elder years. However, one exciting and alternate possibility resides with extending life and continuing the further productive years beyond the standard life cycle.

With extending our livelihood beyond the typical years when we start to slow down, both physically and mentally, we extend our knowledge and experience in contributing to an ever-increasing complex and sophisticated society. Our sense of self-value and continued productive years will prove of greater significance beyond the typical age of retiring.

Extended years also offers individuals the opportunity to expand their current employment prospects, pursue other new career endeavors, continue academic studies, travel, increase financial holdings, and have more productive relationships with family members and friends, especially those who have been fortunate enough to also experience extended life treatments, items that were previously not in the realm of reality.

10

Religious and Spiritual Implications Involving Longevity

There are approximately eighteen major religious groups in America. Thus far, none have presented a hard stance against radical life extension. However, as the topic gains more awareness, some religious groups are taking notice and beginning to voice their concerns from an ethical and religious perspective as it relates to their individual beliefs.

Some religious groups and others reject mainstream medical treatment when they encounter a health problem or injury that would typically necessitate medical intervention. A few of these religious groups include Christian Scientists, Jehovah's Witnesses, Amish, and Scientologists.

There are those individuals and groups who believe primarily on religious grounds that any medical or scientific efforts focused on extending life beyond the natural life cycle (beyond what God has ordained) is unacceptable, repugnant, or even sinful. To the extreme, some of these individuals also believe that attempts to even treat or cure illness during their natural life period is also in violation of their beliefs and therefore remain susceptible to the ailment even unto death.

Pope Benedict XVI (Joseph Ratzinger) expressed concern that dramatically postponing death could end stripping people of their richest experiences, including, among other issues, leaving society in a state of aged paralysis. The pope warned in 2010, "Humanity would become extraordinarily old, there would be no more room for youth and capacity for innovation would die."[248] In 2010, Pope Benedict XVI[249] also spoke against the desire to postpone death indefinitely, warning that endless life on Earth would be no paradise.[250]

Well, life on Earth has never been a paradise, far from it. However, I believe there would be an opportunity to dramatically improve and establish a society that could experience less of the social disparities, improve the environment, live safer and happier lives, and engage in more productive endeavors that would benefit the further progress of humanity.

My optimistic perspective of those living in a radically extended period and living in a vastly different society is based on an expectation that these individuals would retain a uniquely inherent and innate desire and ability to initiate necessary changes that proved evasive before the transition. Of course, this assumes that the population of those living in a radically extended life environment was sufficient in numbers to establish and maintain this new society.

With all due and sincere respect to the pontiff, I see insufficient justification for the pessimistic views held by Pope Benedict, which offers no hope for a better extended life. Granted, if we look to the future of what could be expected by living longer lives. Based upon the historic reality of wars and tormented societies, there could easily be an expectation of simply continuing to exist in the same dismal, disheartened life. Under this perception, one might not be very

[248] Pew Research Center, "To Count Our Days: The Scientific and Ethical Dimensions of Radical Life Extension," https://www.pewforum.org/2013/08/06/to-count-our-days-the scientific-and-ethical-dimensions-of-radical-life-extension.
[249] http://www.vatican.va/holyfather/benedict txvi/homilies/2010/documents/hf ben-xvi hom 20100403 veglia-pasqual en.html.
[250] Pew Research Center, "Living To 120 And Beyond: Americans' Views On Aging, Medical Advances And Radical Life Extension," https://www.pewforum.org/2013/08/06/preface.

enthusiastic about extending their life if, in doing so, they simply continue living with their same downtrodden lifestyle.

Fundamentalists tell us their lives are in the hands of God and we, as physicians, are not God, says Dr. Lorry Frankel, a professor at the Stanford School of Medicine.[251] Consequently, many, especially children, have died from lack of proper and timely professional medical attention. Such is the strength and conviction of these parents.

Such strong religious or related beliefs have and will continue to affect the decisions of individuals who, for themselves, their children, or their invalid, chronically ill parents, not accepting any health-care intervention, no matter how advanced and available such curative lifesaving measures may avail. Therefore, it certainly appears that future advancements within medical science, health care, and technology will only result in the continued rejection by these groups regarding any new and innovative medical applications, even if such advancements can save their lives.

Many individuals do not believe that attempts should be made, especially through draconian intervention, to extend life beyond what would normally be assumed to be the natural end of life. In other words, these individuals believe that to extend the longevity of life for an individual who is near death is assuming the role of God or interfering with the will of God. They further believe that God alone has ordained the time of death for every person.

Of course, there is the other side of the coin that would argue that God has provided the skill and intelligence to medical research scientists and others to bring forth innovative new technologies that can treat, cure, save, and extend lives. But it must be acknowledged that such thinking has also produced advanced weapons of mass destruction that have decimated large populations.

For those who argue that efforts to extend life and avoid death, for any period of time, is interfering with God's plan for our life existence

---

beyond his intent, there were undoubtedly similar attitudes held when life expectancy was limited to an average thirty-five years, then forty-five years, and at other various times to the present day. Thus, such arguments would conclude that God's plan for life expectancy is a variable on a sliding scale.

The point being made here is that God has not imposed limitations upon humanity's creative genius to benefit and advance humankind, which has continued since the caveman discovered the wheel. However, it has certainly proved historically evident that discoveries and inventions intended to improve life for humanity have given way to an opposite intent, yielding more efficient methods to destroy, maim, kill, and impose incredible pain and suffering upon humanity from the earliest time of our existence.

The Soul

The soul, in many religious, philosophical, and mythological traditions, is the incorporeal (lacking material form or substance)[252] essence of a living being.[253] Within the multitude of various religions, cultures, and other beliefs, there are as many different interpretations as to what the soul is and where it is located within the human body. Many believe the soul resides in the brain, while others believe the soul is found within the body at an unknown location, assuming you believe there is a soul. Suffice it for this discussion that we assume the soul is located somewhere inside the human body.

The Spiritual Dilemma

Now, assuming the soul is located within the body, as most believe, a significant dilemma arises when we start to consider extending life by brain transfer or head transplant. This narrative involves two individuals who are participants in the brain transplant procedure.

---

[252] "Incorporeal," The American Heritage Dictionary, Second College Edition.
[253] "Soul," en.wikipedia.org/wiki/Soul.

One individual (the recipient) will retain his head and healthy brain while losing his defective body. The other individual (the donor) will sacrifice his defective head and brain and transfer his healthy body to the recipient.

The Recipient

If we assume the recipient has sacrificed his defective body as a prerequisite to receiving another body from a donor, then his body is obviously dead, it is now a corpse, and we could assume that his soul has departed his physical body. However, if his brain, after the transfer, continues to function and maintains its awareness, how does one reconcile that awareness can continue to exist without the soul, which only departs the body at the time of death? Can a soul exist in an afterlife existence while awareness continues to exist in a post-death environment? What is the disposition of this individual's awareness when at some point in the future the brain ceases to function and becomes brain dead?

No matter how we define death, and there are different criteria, it is typically assumed that once the body (e.g., torso, brain, brain stem, etc.) are deemed to be dead, the soul has departed to an afterlife existence with its pre-death awareness, assuming you believe in an afterlife as I and many others do.

Normally, once the body has died and the soul departs to the afterlife, it is typically assumed by the majority of religious beliefs that the soul brings with it the awareness experienced during its physical life on earth.

The Donor

Relevant to the disposition of the donor's body, it is, in effect, a corpse, absent any viable function since the brain has been severed from it. Thus, at the time of death, it is assumed that the soul has departed the body and the recipient is receiving a corpse without a soul. The donor is transferring his corpse, not his soul, to the recipient. Such a dilemma, in part, further supports the position of those who reject any attempt by current or future medical science to artificially extend life.

However, the above dilemma will not inhibit the efforts of the medical scientific community and their continued research to extend life and awareness by any ethical or religious implication. This is not to suggest that research scientists are emotionally hardened and not sensitive to such non-tangible aspects of their endeavors. If it were not for their continued emphasis, focus, and strong drive to seek new discoveries within their study areas, absent any outside distractions, then little would be accomplished to advance medical achievements for the benefit of humankind.

These scientists do recognize the implication of medical ethics and participate in discussions as to the ethical implications associated within their areas of medical research and investigation. In my opinion, these research scientists will not be inhibited by ethical or religious considerations to the extent that they would de-emphasize the focus of their particular research efforts.

If new advances in medical science were dependent upon approvals by influential outside groups (e.g., ethical, religious, political, legal, etc.), the multitude of subjective and varied opinions could hinder or even eliminate the forward progress so vital to supporting existing and future medical breakthroughs.

11

The Human Aging Process

From the time you were born, the clock has been ticking to your inevitable demise. Aging is such a gradual process that you barely take notice until one day you see something in the mirror that you did not notice before, perhaps a small wrinkle or skin condition. Or maybe you were going through some photos of earlier days and notice yourself as someone who looks a little different now.

This uncomfortable reality can occur at any age, typically beyond the teenage years, and once you become aware of the aging process and its noticeable affects, you will most likely initiate an evaluation of your physical presence throughout most of your remaining life. Oh, for those youthful years of ignorance.

Aging or ageing (spelling differences) in humans is the continued process of changes resulting from predictable diseases caused by the deterioration of our body over time. It is among the most recognized risk factors for most human diseases.[254], [255] Approximately 150,000 people die each day in the world, with about two-thirds (100,000 per day) who die from age-related causes. Industrialized nations have a higher age-related death rate of 90 percent.[256]

---

[254] "Ageing," en.wikipedia.org/wiki/Ageing.
[255] "Life extension," en.wikipedia.org/wiki/Life extension.
[256] "Ageing," en.wikipedia.org/wiki/Ageing.

Currently, there are 962 million people aged sixty and above across the globe, according to the most recent estimates. By the year 2060, this number is projected to more than double, and the number of people aged eighty and above is expected to triple.[257]

Aging is the continued permanent, gradual, and unrelenting physiological cellular decay within the human body that over time will lead to death.[258]

It has been the same unrelenting response by the medical profession and health-care providers, research scientists in various academic and research facilities, the medical device and pharmaceutical industries, and other vested stakeholders that have labored and continue to do so to defeat the conditions that cause or contribute to the aging process, either directly or indirectly.

Some futurists think even more radical changes are coming, including medical treatments that could slow, stop, or even reverse the aging process and allow humans to remain healthy and productive to the age 120 or more, said the report, titled "Living to 120." The possibility that extraordinary life spans could become ordinary life spans no longer seems far-fetched.[259]

Aging of the Brain

Aging is a major risk factor for most common neurodegenerative diseases, including mild cognitive impairment, dementias including Alzheimer's disease, cerebrovascular disease, Parkinson's disease, and Lou Gehrig's disease.[260] The different functions of different tissues in the brain may be more or less susceptible to age-induced

---

[257] C. Paddock, "Brain activity has role in human aging and longevity."

[258] "Ageing," en.wikipedia.org/wiki/Ageing.

[259] L. Collins, "Radical life extension: What would you think of living to 120 and beyond, survey asks," htpps://www.deseret.com/2013/8/6/20523581/radical-life-extension-what-would-you-thinkof-living-to-120-and-beyond-survey-asks#maxine-t-grimm-ag.

[260] "Aging brain," en.wikipedia.org/wiki/Aging brain.

changes. The brain matter can be broadly classified as either gray or white matter.[261]

Brain plasticity refers to the brain's ability to change structure and function. This ties into the common phrase, "If you don't use it, you lose it," which is another way of saying, "If you don't use it, your brain will devote less somatotopic (the organization of the motor areas of the brain and control of the movement of different parts of the body)[262] space for it.[263]

Due to the complexity of the brain, with all of its structures and functions, it is logical to assume that some areas would be more vulnerable to aging than others. Advances in MRI technology have provided the ability to see the brain structure in great detail. Bartzokis et al. has noted that there is a decrease in gray matter volume between adulthood and old age, whereas white matter volume was found to increase from age nineteen to forty and decline after this age.[264]

[261] Id.
[262] "Somatotopic," Medical Dictionary, 27th ed.
[263] "Aging brain," en.wikipedia.org/wiki/Aging brain.
[264] Id.

12

The Aches and Pains of Aging

Walk into any drugstore and find aisles of pain-relieving drugs, roll-ons, and patches allegedly formulated or designed to treat your sore muscles, aching joints, nagging backache, or other pain-related symptoms. The ever-growing, multibillion-dollar pain-relieving industry, especially targeted for the aging population, produces more TV advertisements than any other product.

As we age, it certainly becomes more apparent that our body and physical efforts to perform even the more mundane activities can result in sore, stiff aching muscles and joints, especially in the lower back. The progression of suffering only increases as we advance into the senior years, often with little or no relief despite the promises that constantly pervade TV commercials with claims of instant relief. Such is the natural progression of our human anatomy wearing out as the years pass.

During the early years of human life, especially for women who are often preoccupied with their physical appearance, this has enabled the cosmetic industry to rake in billions of dollars every year by providing an endless line of cosmetic products to appease the millions who desire to improve upon their personal attractiveness.

However, as the years inevitability pass, there comes the time when you begin to notice a recurring pain in your back, hips, neck, or shoulders that you didn't notice before. Gradually these foreboding, bothersome discomforts become more problematic and eventually begin to limit your ability to perform certain activities. Some joint pains become so significant that thousands of patients every year require implantable device replacements for defective hips, knees, spinal area, and other body locations.

While the medical device and pharmaceutical industries are constantly availing more devices and drugs designed and formulated to reduce or even eliminate certain areas of pain, medical research scientists are focused upon correcting the underlining causes of these body abnormalities, including the far more serious ailment such as cancer. Eventually many areas of body pain and suffering will be significantly reduced or even eliminated as scientists conquer the anatomical causes that elicit such pain. However, until that time, the elderly must deal with the uncurable suffering of ailments such as arthritis and other debilitating diseases that dramatically affect the quality of one's life.

I predict that eventually within the foreseeable future, a vast majority of the suffering that the elderly population has continued to endure for centuries will no longer plague humanity. Moreover, I believe that the well-being and health of individuals, especially within the United States, will be so dramatically improved upon that those living in nursing homes and even assisted living facilities will be greatly reduced.

Currently, the elderly population has exploded as the baby boomers have entered their senior years. Thus, the demand for facilities to house so many elderly peoples has resulted in yet further exorbitant fees for those who can afford the unrealistic and unjustified cost to reside in a residence no more elaborate than a typical apartment. And yet these facilities will have little difficulty filling their rental spaces based primarily on availability through supply and demand. While many of these health-care and assisted living facilities do provide some level of medical coverage and support for their residents, the limited extent of such services does not warrant the excessively high cost. While there are justifiable reasons to place certain mental or physically handicapped or debilitating individuals into these facilities, unfortunately too often, they become dumping grounds for elderly family members.

When I was growing up in a row house in Philadelphia, there were three generations living in the same house. It seemed so natural, and I did not fully appreciate how special the experience was until later in life. With my grandparents coming from Europe, this was their culture in that the older family members would be taken care of by their children and continue to live productive lives surrounded by loved ones and fully involved as a family moving forward.

This is no longer the culture in America where now the tendency for many family members is to benevolently, at best, place their aging parents into a storage facility. I speculate that within the foreseeable future, there will be no need to have patients and family members placed on life support, sometimes for extended periods of time, while the patient and family members endure the agonizing and inevitable wait for the patient's demise.

The primary cause of death involving the elderly will be natural causes associated with the deterioration of one's body and mind within the normal life span of humans and lacking many of the pre-death suffering ailments as currently endured by terminally ill patients in hospice care. Death, for the majority, will no longer involve sustained artificial life existence and traumatic, long-drawn-out suffering, but rather a more peaceful and humane life-terminating experience.

Olshansky et al. have opined,

> even eliminating all aging-related causes of death currently written on the death certificates of the elderly population will not increase human life expectancy by more than 15 years. In order for this limit to be exceeded, the underlying processes of aging that increase vulnerability to all common causes of death currently appearing on death certificates will have to be modified.

In my opinion, when all the causes of death written on death certificates are eliminated, as expressed by Olshansky[265] et al., who

---

[265] S. Olshansky et al., "Position Statement on Human Aging," https://academic. oup.com/biomedgerontology/article/57/8/B292/556758.

believe the end result will provide no more than fifteen extra years of life expectancy, this represents a significant number of additional years not to be snide upon as a trivial accomplishment. I believe that most, if not all, causes of death involving senior citizens will be eliminated in our lifetime, meaning within the next twenty-five to fifty years.

While scientific medical research continues to reduce or eliminate causes that contribute to the aging process and elderly deaths, parallel research programs focused on extending life are also moving forward in an aggressive manner.

When Does Aging Become Apparent?

The answer is dependent upon a number of factors, including your race, lifestyle, heritage, exposure to the sun, general health, and so forth. For Caucasian women, it's typically around the late thirties when fine lines on the forehead and around the eyes become noticeable. For women of color, these skin-aging signs occur ten years more slowly than for Caucasians.[266]

In your thirties, your body's metabolism starts slowing. Around forty, the natural life cycle of skin cells is stopped, and it could affect your complexion in many ways. During the early fifties, the skin barrier function weakens, which makes skin dry and unable to retain enough hydration on its own. In your sixties, all the aging processes dramatically accelerate.[267] Humans typically reach their prime physical and mental ability during their twenties and thirties.

There are seven primary signs of aging. These include fine lines and wrinkles. (Fine lines, crow's feet, and wrinkles are the most evident and often most concern-causing signs of aging for men and women.) Other signs are dullness of skin as the glowing, dewy skin of youth slowly fades with age, uneven skin tone, dry skin tone,

---

[266] G. Gold, "This Is the Age When You Start to Visibly Look Older," https://www.marieclaire.com/beauty/news/a16636/the-age-when-aging-begins.
[267] Id.

blotchiness and age spots, rough skin texture, and visible pores.[268] Of course, there are other signs of premature aging, including sunspots caused by years of sun exposure, gaunt hands, sagging skin, and hair loss, and so forth.

Dermatologists offer the following ways to reduce premature skin aging:

1. Protect your skin from the sun every day.
2. Apply self-tanner rather than get a tan.
3. Stop smoking.
4. Avoid repetitive facial expressions.
5. Eat a healthy, well-balanced diet.
6. Drink less alcohol.
7. Exercise most days of the week.
8. Cleanse your skin gently.
9. Wash your face twice a day and after sweating heavily.
10. Apply a facial moisturizer every day.
11. Stop using skin care products that sting or burn.[269]

Age-related deterioration is due largely to the complex and numerous forms of damage that occur over time to the macromolecules, such as DNA, proteins, and lipids, that make up our bodies.[270]

Characteristics associated with aging are experienced by most humans during the span of their life. A few examples include:

1. In the mid-twenties, female fertility declines.[271]
2. The human body mass is decreased after age thirty until age seventy years, and muscles do not have the ability to respond

---

[268] "The seven signs of ageing," https://platinumdermatology.com.au/articles/the-seven-signs-of-ageing.
[269] G. Gold, "This Is the Age When You Start to Visibly Look Older."
[270] J. Herbert, "The Science of Replacement as a Means of Escaping Aging," blogs.einstein.yu.edu/the-science-of-replacement-as-a-means-of-escaping-aging.
[271] "Ageing," en.wikipedia.org/wiki/Ageing.

to exercise, with the loss of muscle mass and strength being a common factor.

3. At about age fifty, the hairs start turning gray. Partial and continued hair loss also typically starts at about age fifty and affects about 30 to 50 percent of males and about 25 percent of females.[272]

4. Between ages forty-four and fifty-eight, menopause typically occurs.

5. Between the ages of sixty to sixty-four, the level of osteoarthritis rises to about 53 percent.[273]

6. Over the age of seventy-five, people experience hearing loss that inhibits their ability to effectively communicate.

7. More than 50 percent of Americans have a cataract or have had cataract surgery by the age of eighty.

8. About 25 percent of those over eighty-five become frail and experience decreased strength, diminished physical activity, and lack of energy.

9. Between the ages of sixty-five and seventy-four years, about 3 percent of people will experience dementia with approximately 50 percent of those over eighty-five years of age losing their intellectual abilities due to impairment of memory.

10. Over the age of eighty, approximately 12 percent of people will suffer macular degeneration, causing loss of vision that will continue to increase with age.

11. As the brain ages, intelligence declines and drops abruptly as people near the end of life. After the age twenty, there is about a 10 percent decline with each decade in the brain's myelinated (myelin sheath) axons (the process of a neuron by which impulses travel).[274], [275]

---

[272] Id.

[273] Id.

[274] "Myelin sheath," Medical Dictionary, 27th ed.

[275] "Ageing," en.wikipedia.org/wiki/Ageing.

As with most things in life that require periodic maintenance and replacement of damaged parts, so too does the human body. With the increase in life expectancy over time, the adverse effects upon the body, as illustrated above, should also decrease proportionally.

The rare exception to the term *successful aging* was first recognized in the 1950s, where it was defined as "having the absence of physical and cognitive disabilities." Rowe and Kahn defined successful aging in their 1987 article as "retaining three components: 1. Freedom from disease and disability, 2. high cognitive and physical functioning; and 3. social and productive engagement."[276]

---

[276] Id.

13

Fighting the Aging Process

The antiaging industry has provided several hormone therapies. However, such treatments have been viewed, especially by the American Medical Association, as potentially dangerous and lacking demonstrated effectiveness.[277]

Antiaging products have been a very lucrative worldwide industry. They market their supplements and hormone products in such a manner to emphasize slowing or even reversing the aging process. However, many of these claims have not been supported or validated by any approving organization, like the FDA.

For example, in 2009, in the U.S. market, the industry generated roughly $50 billion in revenue. No doubt, any advertised product that makes such claims will have a significant population of consumers all too willing to buy their products even though many of these products have not been proven to be either safe or effective by the FDA.[278] Leonard Hayflick et al. have also criticized the antiaging industry and their dealings as unscrupulous profiteering in their sale of unproven antiaging supplements.[279]

Most individuals purchase antiaging products in an attempt to ward off the inevitable and ever-present appearance of aging skin.

---

[277] "Life extension," en.wikipedia.org/wiki/Life extension.

[278] Id.

[279] Id.

The most prolific cause of perceived premature skin aging is the result of overexposure to the sun, as previously discussed, with its harmful and even deadly radiation.

The Problem

The leading cause of death in the United States involves the cardiovascular system. The most common change in the cardiovascular system is the stiffening of the blood vessels and arteries, causing your heart to work harder to pump blood through them. The heart muscles change to adjust to the increased workload. Your heart rate at rest will stay about the same, but it won't increase during activities as much as it used to. These changes increase the risk of high blood pressure (hypertension) and other cardiovascular problems.[280]

You can do the following: Include physical activity in your daily routine. Eat a healthy diet. Don't smoke.

There has been a resurgence and proliferation of advertisers and entrepreneurs who have been promoting antiaging and lifestyle-enhancing products that, in some cases, go as far as to claim their products will slow, stop, or even reverse the process of aging. Even though in most cases there is little or no scientific basis for these claims, the public continues to spend vast sums of money on these products and their alleged lifestyle improvements, some of which may actually be harmful.[281]

I have noticed certain aging products advertised on TV (cannot identify for obvious reasons) that in my estimations will provide an immediate improvement to the aging problem identified; however, the active ingredients that produce an apparent immediate improvement will only last for a limited time. The longer-term effects can be potentially hazardous, especially with continued use, and

---

[280] Mayo Foundation for Education and Research (MFMER), "Aging: What to expect."
[281] S. Olshansky et al., "Position Statement on Human Aging."

result in creating a condition more dramatic and problematic than initially identified.

Next time you watch TV, take notice of the number of commercials and the claims provided by the product manufacturers of anti-aging products. Also, include any cosmetic products that also include ingredients that can prove harmful, especially with extended use. Most viewers simply accept that products advertised on TV will deliver on their promises without any concerns. However, as a forensic examiner and investigator, I can assure you that often such products do not live up to their promises and can potentially result in serious injuries to the user or patient.

Again, even with those products that you perceive as being innocuous, I strongly recommend that you read the package inserts, if available, and the labeling on the package cover. Remember, these manufacturers want to sell their products, and often they will not provide you with full disclosure details, especially pertaining to warnings and precautions as required pursuant to FDA regulations and the law. For those of you who would be particularly cautious, call the FDA to discover their position on the particular product and determine what level of FDA clearance, if any, they provided for the subject product before the manufacturer was authorized to release it into commercial distribution.

Moreover, keep this in mind pertaining to any drug, device, or cosmetic product you may have purchased or received through any health-care provider and subsequently experienced a concern involving its use. The FDA has promulgated (as required by law) and by law pursuant to the Federal Food, Drug, and Cosmetic (FD&C) Act very stringent regulations that require any health-related concern to be reported to the Agency. These notifications to the FDA are called complaints reports and are taken very seriously by the FDA and thoroughly investigated by them. These complaint reports are a matter of public record and available to all citizens for review. I again strongly recommend that any product regulated by the FDA that has appeared to have caused you or a family member a concern, you utilize the full services the FDA provides to you in order to determine if the subject product has performed in a safe, effective, and reliable manner and in response to its specified formulation or design intent. These recommendations are particularly significant as they pertain to drugs, both prescribed and over-the-counter, and medical devices, especially any implantable device.

Here's an example: I have investigated a large number of alleged defective implantable medical devices that have caused or contributed to a serious injury or death [e.g., cardiovascular pacemakers, defibrillators, drug dispensers, and orthopedic devices (e.g., hip, knee, spinal, etc.)] and many other implantable devices. Manufacturers of all medical products must maintain complaint files and are responsible and required to evaluate each complaint, pursuant to the specific areas identified within the regulations.

One of the initial requirements under regulations is for the product manufacturer to determine whether the reported incident must then be forwarded to the FDA. The information reported must include a determination of the following minimal details: whether the device failed to meet specifications, whether the device was being used for treatment or diagnosis; the relationship, if any, of the device to the reported incident or adverse event; the name of the device; the date the complaint was received; any unique device identification; the name, address, and phone number of the complainant; the nature and details of the complaint; the dates and results of the investigation; any corrective action taken; and any reply to the complainant.[282]

When I begin my investigation of a particular product (and I have investigated many hundreds of different medical devices and drugs for causes involving a serious injury or death), I am often surprised at the large number of reported adverse incidents. This is a significant issue when attempting to identify the cause(s) and areas of responsibility and accountability.

Now, if the manufacturer determined that the reported incident must be forwarded to the FDA with responses to the above specific

---

[282] Code of Federal Regulations (CFR). Food & Drugs. Parts 800-1299. Revised April 1, 2017. Part 820.198 - Complaint Files.

areas of concern and other details, the manufacturer must identify and provide, at minimum, the alleged cause of the patient's serious injury or death. Factors that may have caused or contributed to a patient's serious injury or death would include events occurring as a result of failure, malfunction, improper or inadequate design, manufacture, labeling, or user error.[283]

I have emphasized the above so you can appreciate the significant amount of critical data and information available to you online and through the FDA under the Freedom of Information Act that will pertain to any medical or drug product that has potentially caused you or a family member to be concerned about a perceived injury or, worse, the use of the product.

Once you gain access to the adverse incident reports, also referred to as medical device reports (MDRs), pertaining to submitted complaint reports, you will be able to determine if similar issues related to your specific concern have been previously reported and how many were reported over an extended period of time. In some cases, you may actually determine that your area of concern may warrant contacting an attorney to determine if you have a viable case worthy of legal action.

---

[283] Id. Part 803-Medical Device Reporting. Subpart 803.3c (1)-(6).

14

Drugs That Help Us to Live Longer

The ten most important drugs in history have been identified as follows: penicillin (1938), insulin (1922), aspirin (1899), smallpox vaccine (1798), morphine (1827), ether (1846), chemotherapy drugs (1956), HIV protease inhibitors (1995), Botox (1978), and warfarin.[284] The ten most prescribed drugs and their brand names include atorvastatin (Lipitor), levothyroxine (Synthroid), lisinopril (Prinivil, Zestril), gabapentin (Neurontin), amlodipine (Norvasc), hydrocodone/ acetaminophen (Vicodin, Norco), amoxicillin (Amoxil), omeprazole (Prilosec), metformin (Glucophage), and losartan (Cozaar).[285] Bill Gifford reported,

> There are some promising hints of antiaging properties involving the diabetes drug Metformin, which FDA approved in 2015 for clinical trial. If it helps more of us live healthy lives up to the ceiling of 120 years, that would be welcome progress.[286]

---

[284] B. Lau, "10 most important medicines in history," MIMS Today.

[285] A. Paavola, "10 most prescribed drugs in the U.S. in Q1. (2019)," https://www. bechershospitalreview.com/pharmacy/10-most-prescribed-drugs-in-the-u-s-in-q1.html.

[286] M. Shermer, "Radical Life-Extension Is Not Around the Corner," https://www. newscientist.com/article/radical-life-extension-is-not-around-the-corner.

Metformin is an everyday remedy taken to treat type 2 diabetics. A recent study has indicated that metformin may also function as a longevity drug, indicating that diabetics prescribed this drug were less likely to die than those using other drugs. Moreover, about 15 percent were less likely to die than people without diabetes who did not take metformin.[287]

Subsequent to the release of metformin, there were eight recent discoveries involving additional health benefits provided by taking metformin: improved male fertility, improved female fertility, longer life span, colon cancer prevention and treatment, prostate cancer treatment, ovarian cancer treatment, enhanced gut bacteria, and dementia prevention.[288] What we didn't know until recently is how many additional benefits researchers would discover for metformin that aren't related to diabetes, leading many to wonder if metformin is the Holy Grail.

Therefore, if you currently have type 2 diabetics and have been prescribed metformin, consider yourself fortunate to receive the additional treatment that now appears to function as a drug to extend life as well. However, this anticipated aging benefit of metformin has not yet been approved by the FDA for this expanded use.

Most of these drugs will control or eliminate the affliction for which they are prescribed and thereby further extend the life of the individual. While these drugs have been specifically formulated to treat certain body functions, organs, and systems, they also provide a secondary antiaging capability, not often appreciated by the recipient.

There are also specific drugs and research topics targeted to slow the aging process currently being studied. One research study focuses on the effects of a calorie restriction diet, which has demonstrated its effect to extending the life of some animals.[289]

---

[287] C. Wilson, "Everyday drugs could give extra years of life," https://www.newscientist.com/article/mg22429894-000-everyday-drugs-could-give-extra-years-of-life.

[288] S. Orrange, "8 Surprising Benefits of Metformin Besides Treating Diabetes," Good Rx, Inc.

[289] "Life extension," en.wikipedia.org/wiki/Life extension.

Some drugs that have already been approved by the FDA for other intended uses are now being studied in animals for potential longevity effects. These drugs include Rapamycin, metformin, Geroprotectors, MitoQ, Resveratrol, and Pterostilbene (drug 4, 5, and 6) are dietary supplements.[290]

A major cause of disease and death is the aging of the immune system. It is why older people are more susceptible to infection and why they normally have a weaker response to vaccines.[291] Common drugs like low-dose aspirin and statins are typically taken by healthy people to reduce the risk of heart disease. Animal studies have indicated that both these drugs extend life span and retain anti-inflammatory effects.[292]

While some drugs have the potential to extend life by a few years, the pharmaceutical industry wants to focus on the development of drugs targeted specifically to extending life. However, getting such drugs approved by the FDA as a treatment for specific age-related conditions could prove difficult because the FDA does not currently recognize aging as a medical condition that requires treatment.[293]

---

[290] Id.
[291] C. Wilson, "Everyday drugs could give extra years of life," https://www.newscientist.com/article/mg22429894-000-everyday-drugs-could-give-extra-years-of-life.
[292] Id.
[293] Id.

15

Perception vs. Reality

The perception of one's personal characteristics may not be based on the reality of whom they are, especially as others perceive them. Many factors, both physiological and neurological, can cause or contribute to an inaccurate perception or interpretation of who you are. Furthermore, the reality of who you are would most likely be inaccurately described by others who presume to know you, even by your closest family members and friends.

Such differences within the perception (or description) of an individual can be demonstrated by first recording how one would fully describe their personal characteristics and then have family members and friends record their perception or interpretation of the individual's characteristics. In most cases, it would soon become apparent that there exists a variation in how others perceive the individual, based on their own perceptions and interpretations.

Therefore, everyone has their own perception of their own reality pertaining to who they believe they are. As such, it must be assumed therefore that any such perception cannot be assumed to be a reality since the factors required to validate the individual reality cannot be effectively and accurately accomplished.

Perception depends on our five basic senses to facilitate our ability to identify a familiar friend in a crowd or recognize the scent of a flower. Our perceptions are formed from our prior learning experiences that will influence how we will ultimately perceive and interpret our environment and our interaction within our environment.

Based upon how individual perceptions have been formed from an early time in life, there will ultimately be occasions when disagreements will arise because in many situations, there will be different interpretations based on our individual perceptions and prior experiences that may generate a dispute or argument as to the issue at hand.

So what does perception versus reality have to do with extending life? Well, quite a lot actually. For example, I discussed the current health hazards that may pertain to you, in part or in whole. The individual health hazards are realities in your life. How you perceive these individual hazardous circumstances in your life and, more importantly, how you respond to your perceptions will determine if you ultimately extend or shorten your life.

16

The Five Human Senses

In normal everyday life, we subconsciously depend on our five primary senses to enable our activities and perceive through the unique capability of each sense our environment and how to respond accordingly. These five basic senses include sight, smell, hearing, taste, and touch and have evolved to effectively communicate information specific to each sense to the brain for processing and response.

Sense organs are defined as specialized organs that help to perceive the world around us. They are an integral part of our lives and the only way that enables us to appropriately and accurately perceive our environment. Some neurologists believe there are more than five senses, numbering from nine to twenty-one. These include things like perception of heat, pressure, pain, and balance, among others.[294]

Each of the five basic senses provides a unique and critical link of information perceived by each sense of its surroundings and sent to the brain. The brain processes the information received and communicates to the body the action believed to be appropriate. For example, "I want to take a right turn at the next intersection." This does not infer that the response produced by the brain was

---

[294] D. Wood, "The Five Senses & Their Functions," https://www.study.com/academy/lesson/the-five-senses-their-functions.html.

the appropriate action to take as being right or wrong. The brain is communicating responsive information based on what has been previously stored from prior experience.

Without previously stored information, the brain may not be able to respond accordingly. For example, "I have not been to this intersection before, so I'm not sure which way I should turn. I'm lost." It's not quite that simplistic, but the point is made.

Without these five basic senses, our brain and thus our body would be unable to function properly or effectively. Many individuals can and do live productive lives absent one or even more of these five senses (e.g., sight or hearing). However, the ability of all our senses produces our awareness and thus, to this extent, defines life.

17

HOW can I Exist Beyond my normal life span?

Currently a number of anticipated but speculative alternatives sometime in the future may offer to the elderly and terminally ill a process and/or mechanism of preserving the body (e.g., corpse) or head (e.g., brain) until some future time when science and medicine have advanced to a point where it is theoretically possible, although highly unlikely, to revive the corpse and brain or, by other means, transfer the brain and/or its awareness to a suspension solution, computer, or artificial housing mechanism (e.g., robot).

Cryogenics

One currently available but highly dubious process is cryogenics, which has been around since 1967 when the first person was cryonically frozen. Some companies advertise and propose attempts to extend a person's life beyond their physical death through the cryogenics process. People have their body or head cryogenically frozen once they have been diagnosed with a terminal illness, like cancer, and declared legally dead. Some cryogenic companies even claim that their clients will keep their personality, including their memories, knowledge, and experience.

It is the hope of those who are subjected to the cryogenics deep freeze that in the future, scientists will develop a method to revitalize the body (cells and tissue) and the cognitive pre-cryogenics capabilities of the brain and bring them back to life when there may be a cure for their terminal illness.

Those who voluntarily chose to have their corpse placed in a cryonics chamber are waiting and anticipating a cure not currently available to them. Approximately 350 people throughout the world have elected to participate in this experimental deep-freeze process. However, scientists and physicians do not currently have the understanding required to reanimate a frozen body or brain.[295]

One expert believes that a corpse could possibly be reanimated within the next ten years.[296] Such unrealistic claims are void of any support from mainstream science and pose a potentially dangerous influence on people considering the cryogenics process in their future.

Although there are those who believe in the experimental process of cryogenically deep freezing the human body and brain, there are strong opposing opinions by the medical profession and medical research scientists. Many experts in related fields believe there is no chance of successfully recovering frozen cells and tissue. They cite examples like the heart and kidneys that have never been successfully thawed, not including any consideration for the vulnerability of other organs and systems that would be involved in the deep-freeze process.

Such experts believe that once the body and brain have been frozen, as in the process of cryogenics, irreversible damage has occurred, rendering any possibility of a successful recovery impossible.[297] Medical experts say once cells are damaged during freezing and

---

[295] H. Pettit, "First human frozen by cryogenics could be brought back to life 'in just TEN years', claims expert," https://www.dailymail.co.uk/sciencetech/article-5270257/Cryogenics-corpses-brought-10-years.html.
[296] Id.
[297] Id.

turned to mush, they cannot be converted back to living tissue, any more than you can turn a scrambled egg back into a raw whole egg.[298]

Although cryonics is legal in several countries, a human body (a corpse) or brain cannot be cryogenically frozen until the person is declared legally dead. As such, when a future attempt is made to resuscitate the corpse and/or brain, the person would still be legally dead with a death certificate to validate their death. So the logical question would be: if the corpse or brain were successfully revived, would they be issued a new birth certificate? What governing documents would identify their state of existence?

It is not possible for a corpse to be reanimated after undergoing vitrification (ultra-rapid freezing), as this causes damage to the brain, including its neural network.[299] Such a highly controversial procedure has never been proven to actually work, and it is far more likely that it cannot and will not ever be determined as a viable, safe, and effective procedure.

Yevgeny Aleksandrov, PhD in physical and mathematical science and the head of the RAS commission, which challenges pseudoscience, has stated that in his opinion, "Cryonics is a purely commercial exploitation of the dream of an afterlife. It is impossible to prove experimentally that the ideas of the cryonists are possible and no one has learned how to revive a cryogenic corpse yet."[300]

The entire field of cryonics is not regulated by any agency. For example, the FDA with their congressional-mandated responsibility to assure that only safe and effective medical devices, drugs, and experimental procedures are permitted, has not authorized any clinical studies involving the subject process and will not be able to do so until a future proponent can assemble justifiable data and evidence to warrant their involvement, which in my opinion would be near impossible to accomplish.

---

[298] Id.

[299] "Cryonics," en.wikipedia.org.wiki/Cryonics.

[300] Y. Aleksandrov, "Between life and death: how to freeze yourself and wake up in future," https://medium.com/cryogen/between-life-and-death-how-to-freeze-yourself-and-wake-up-in-future-1ff8715abf80.

The probability of obtaining future authorization from FDA to conduct clinical studies involving a cryogenic corpse is not conceivable based on the agency's stringent prerequisite requirements to justify the study. Moreover, the cryonics experimental procedure could not be approved for clinical study because, if for no other reason, it would involve an attempt to freeze and subsequently recover a legally declared dead person (e.g., their corpse) and their brain.

There is no authorization by Congress for FDA or any other organization to participate in any form of research or inquiry that would recognize the viable and justifiable process of freezing a human corpse and brain with the primary intent of reviving them sometime in the future in order to reestablish life and awareness. Dead tissue and cells remain dead and cannot be restored to the level of their pre-death condition.

Admittedly, history and science have taught us that the term *never* has often been proved inaccurate. However, based on today's insights, it would be accurate to believe that there will not be any acceptable procedure in the foreseeable future to successfully reanimate a corpse or brain, especially with the current methods of cryonic deep freezing.

There has yet to be, and it is highly doubtful, that any safe and effective prescribed process nor any viable foreseeable process to safely and effectively prep either the brain or corpse to enhance some higher level of potential success during the reanimation recovery process. Moreover, the future probability for either to be reanimated would be near impossible to accomplished to the extent of the pre-cryopreserved body and brain level functions. There is simply no possibility of raising a legally declared dead person (e.g., no Lazarus rising).

The requirements to prepare a corpse or brain safely and effectively for a future attempt at reanimation are not on any horizon within the scientific community or currently worthy of any scientific pursuit. There simply is no sufficient foundation of data and discovery to warrant such a speculative endeavor. There is only unsubstantial and unqualified speculation as to how reanimation of a corpse or brain could occur with countless unanswered questions. It is especially significant to dismiss any expectation that the brain could reestablish conscience thought (awareness).

Current methods of preparing a corpse for deep freeze are limited to solutions that attempt to maintain a certain temperature within the corpse, designed to protect the corpse from damage during the cryonics process, making sure that ice crystals do not form, which could damage the cells and tissue.[301]

However, such minimal preservation attempts barely touch on appropriate considerations and difficulties to be resolved for all the other body and brain functions in order to anticipate (hope for) a safe and effective recovery.

Perfusion of these "cryoprotectants" involves a complex process that must be initiated at the earliest opportunity within the first day of death, after which the corpse is immersed in liquid nitrogen at -196 degrees Celsius.[302]

It is very improbable that a human body (corpse) or brain from a severed head could be successfully revived, even in the distant future, but if it did occur, then what follow-up expectation would there be for what happens next with either? Would all the frozen organs and systems, including the central nervous system in the corpse, function in the same or similar manner as before they were placed in a cryonic deep freeze? Definitely not!

However, let us imagine that such a recovery process was possible. What would the reanimated brain theoretically experience? If the brain were indeed to somehow awaken without the ability of physical sensation or to speak, hear, or see, what would it most likely experience? Imagine the prospect of suddenly becoming aware of your existence in a sensory void environment with the worst prolonged experience of fear imaginable.

There would be no ability to experience any cognitive or sensory sensation. The awakened brain would be unable to communicate in any manner what it is feeling or if it were suffering physically or

---

[301] Id.
[302] Id.

psychologically. The revived brain could literally exist in the worst imaginable hell with no possibility to self-impose relief or even the termination of its awareness. I wonder how this topic was presented to those who were considering the deep-freeze process and how it was addressed in their consent form and contract. Therefore, the goal of reanimation, if we assume it were possible to achieve, cannot and should not be attempted without the availability and assurance of some anticipated level of cognitive reasoning and comprehension after the reanimation procedure, which would be near impossible to verify.

Having concluded that any realistic expectation of such possible recovery or resurrection should remain in the realm of science fiction, it certainly is understandable that those who have participated in this deep-freeze process realized that the only other alternative was death and, regardless of all the skepticism, believed that some hope for a future existing awareness is better than none. The first body to be cryogenically frozen was in 1967 and is the only body frozen before 1974 and remains preserved today.[303]

Again, the process cannot be initiated until the patient has been declared legally dead and must take place at the very earliest opportunity, ideally within the first two minutes and no longer than fifteen minutes from the time the heart has stopped.[304], [305]

Josh Bocanegra, CEO of Humai's, a fairly recent start-up venture, claims that he wants to transfer your consciousness to an artificial body so you can live forever.[306] Bocanegra explains how he cryogenically intends to do this. "We're using artificial intelligence and nanotechnology to store data of conversational styles, behavioral

---

[303] "Cryonics," en.wikipedia.org/wiki/Cryonics.
[304] H. Pettit, "First human frozen by cryogenics could be brought back to life 'in just TEN years', claims expert." 1
[305] F. MacDonald, "A New Start-Up Wants to Transfer Your Consciousness to an Artificial Body So You Can Live Forever," https://www.sciencealert.com/a-new-start-up-wants-to-transfer-your-consciousness-to-an-artificial-body-so-you-can-live-forever.
[306] Id.

patterns, thought processes and information about how your body functions from the inside out."[307]

These data will be coded into multiple sensor technologies, which will be built into an artificial body with the brain of a deceased human. Using cloning technology, we will restore the brain as it matures. Bocanergra further explains that while it sounds very much like the singularity (with our brains being uploaded into computers), basically the company just wants to cryogenically freeze your brain and put it back in another body once the technology is ready to hook it up and repair it.[308] When the technology is fully developed, we'll implant the brain into an artificial body.[309]

Not a surprise that Bocanegra has been unable to secure any venture capital for his dubious expectations to reanimate a stored cryogenically frozen brain and implant the revived brain into an artificial body. The can't-do reasons why Bocanegra's intentions to accomplish his procedure, as described previously, are so numerous and formidable that it borders on the realm of fanciful thinking, unrealistic expectations, and with the eventual reality dawning on Bocanerga that he should redirect his talents into other more profitable ventures.

So is cryonics worthy of viable and justifiable consideration for extending one's life? No! After reviewing all available and extensive data, opinions, and discussions on this highly controversial subject and considering both sides of contention, it is my concluding opinion that the cryonics process of deep freezing a body or brain with the intent and belief that the dead tissue and cells can somehow be reanimated in the future when anticipated curative medicine or procedure is available will not result in the extended life of the individual or reestablish awaken awareness. Dead cells and tissue will remain dead.

Scientists generally are hugely skeptical that this kind of preservation will ever work. Dr. Ken Hayworth, a neuroscientist

---

[307] Id.
[308] Id.
[309] Id.

at the Howard Hughes Medical Institute in Virginia, was an early enthusiast for cryonics and had arranged to be frozen upon his death. However, his research led him to suspect that the cryonic freezing process damaged brains so badly that revival was impossible. He concluded that a lot of these companies were selling false hope. This led him to abandon his cryonics contract.[310]

There are acceptable and proven effective methods of cryogenics involving tissue specimens, sperm, and eggs that are routinely frozen for medical and research uses. However, in the end, cryonics is similar to the endless discussion about the existence of UFOs on TV, movies, and books. But where is the real hands-on undeniable proof or evidence to support such strong assertions? There simply is none. Although advocates on both topics aggressively push their narrative, there remains only unsupported speculation.

Science and medicine have maintained that dead tissue cannot be brought back to life. Dead is dead and will always remain dead. There exists far more scientific data and research findings that conclude frozen tissue and cells cannot be reclaimed for any reanimated physical or neurological expectation.

And yet it must be acknowledged that there are those who believe so strongly in the possibility of cryonics that they have invested heavily in their time, efforts, and funding to either establish facilities to perform the process or support the belief that cryonics will produce future successful results during and after the reanimation process. There are even cryonics conventions.

Initial attempts to preserve and store a corpse were performed in the 1960s and early 1970s, which ended in failure.[311] As of 2014, about 250 corpses have been cryogenically preserved in the United States, and around 1,500 people have signed up to have their remains preserved.[312] In 2016, four facilities could supposedly cryogenically

---

[310] K. Hayworth, "Preserving your brain might kill you, but it could help you live forever," https://www.cbc.ca/radio/quirks/may-5-2018-preserving-brains-for-uploading-coral-reefs-sound-sick-south-american-child-sacrifice-and-more-1.46470.
[311] "Cryonics," en.wikipedia.org.wiki/Cryonics.
[312] Id.

preserve a corpse with the intent of reanimation in the future, three in the United States and one in Russia. However, as of 2018, all but one of the pre-1973 cryonic companies have gone out of business and subsequently defrosted their stored corpses and disposed of them.[313] This concluding reality is certainly not the message enthusiastically conveyed to prospective clients of cryonic firms.

In 2018, start-up Nectome announced it had developed a method to preserve the human brain until the date that advanced scanning methods are practical. Only one issue: "It has to be fresh." That is, you have to be alive when they do the process, which kills you.[314]

Nectome CEO Robert McLntyre believes in his technology, pitching it as a way to save your precious memories rather than create a full digital simulacrum (an image or representation of something)[315] of your consciousness. Over thirty people have put down $10,000 deposits to be on the list for preservation.[316]

Therefore, in all fairness, the jury cannot render a definitive verdict until such time when the cryonics process is determined to be successful or, as I predict, remain unsuccessful. In the meantime, I hold to my opinion that scientists have concluded appropriately that cryonics cannot restore dead cells or tissue to their prior state of living, viable cells, and tissue.

---

[313] Id.

[314] K. Jensen, "Will We Ever Be Able to Upload Our Brains?" https://www.pcmag.com/news/will-we-ever-be-able-to-upload-our-brains.

[315] "Simulacrum," The American Heritage Dictionary, Second College Edition.

[316] K. Jensen, "Will We Ever Be Able to Upload Our Brains?"

18

Pre-clinical Trials

Prior to considering clinical studies involving humans, responsible medical device facilities and clinical investigators also want to determine in advance of human trials if any unidentified adverse issues, especially pertaining to potential risks and hazards, can be identified and responded to in an appropriate manner. For procedures involving human head transplantation, the list of potential serious risk factors is certainly formidable.

Until appropriate and adequate data have been accumulated through animal studies and other areas of research focus to justify moving forward with human clinical trials involving head transplants or brain transfers, and until the specified target objectives have been successfully accomplished, it would be vastly premature and extremely hazardous to attempt such a highly problematic procedure.

Pertaining to the head-to-body transplant, some of the material components anticipated to be included in the procedure, such as implantable orthopedic hardware, may have already been cleared or approved by the FDA through previous animal studies and/or other human clinical studies to validate their intended usage and therefore have been determined to be safe, effective, and reliable for those other intended uses.

However, since a head-to-body transfer would involve such a radical and entirely new realm of surgical procedure, the FDA would undoubtedly require new data governed by existing and new agency regulations for clinical studies to justify that the existing devices and related procedure could be accomplished safely and effectively for head-to-body transplants.

Again, in my opinion, this is an unrealistic expectation and indeed would doubtfully not reach any viable or serious contemplation of such a radical surgical procedure, at least not until some distant time when such data can be obtained and validated, if ever.

The pre-clinical animal studies involving head-to-body transplantation would be such an incomprehensible surgical procedure to the outside world that animal welfare boards and other animal protection groups would feel such disdain and revolt over their interpretation and conception of the procedure that they would vehemently oppose animals being subjected to such a hideous surgical procedure, reminiscent of science-fiction movies like *Frankenstein*. Moreover, they would certainly obtain the support of the public to forcefully prohibit any such studies involving animals.

The pre-clinical concerns of using animals would be potentially problematic for the investigators involving head-to-body transplantation. Point of fact, attempting to obtain approval to conduct animal studies represents only the beginning of a long road of barriers and continued frustrations for the sponsor and their clinical investigators.

Based on my prior experience working with critical, high-risk implantable medical devices and their associated surgical procedures, the anticipated regulatory requirements and law that must be addressed are truly staggering and overwhelming to the extent that I cannot conceive any opportunity within the foreseeable or even distant future, for a sponsor to successfully accomplish clinical studies that would produce adequate data to justify FDA scrutiny and subsequent approval of the proposed surgical procedure.

Looking through current lenses, there simply is no observable pathway to introducing any methodology or protocol that would justify a human head-to-body transplant procedure. This, I anticipate, will prove to be the devastating reality that awaits the sponsor and clinical investigators who may one day in the distant future realize that all attempts to accomplish a safe and effective surgical procedure to transplant a head to a body would result in complete failure. Although there are some scientists who firmly believe that the human head-to-body transplantation will occur, I just do not see it happening.

However, having said that, my opinion can only be based upon my interpretation of existing accomplishments within the neuroscience field of research and all other related fields of study, including realistic and justifiable speculations as to future potential accomplishment that can only be viewed through lenses that do not provide any clarity of what awaits future accomplishments. As stated earlier, science has taught us, "Never say never."

19

The Critical Decision

Imagine you are dying and yet you have a sound mind and clarity of thought. Due to the cause of your physical abnormality or disease, your brain and your awareness are about to be sacrificed due to a terminal illness or because a vital organ can no longer provide its support function to your continued life since it is failing. Thus, your life awareness of existence, your surroundings, and your thinking process, will terminate at the moment your body is no longer capable of supporting your cognitive capabilities and you die.

Now, under the previous assumptions, let us further imagine that you are visited by a neurology research scientist who informs you that a new, highly innovative research project has availed the possibility that your awareness, your thinking process, and your memory can continue beyond your current life expectancy if the newly proposed experimental procedure proved successful.

Moreover, since it has been determined that you have no apparent neurological defects and are mentally sound with all the necessary cognitive capabilities, prerequisites, and fully functional senses, you have been deemed a viable candidate to participate in a new neurological clinical transplant study, should you decide to do so. However, potential candidates for head, brain, and even the donor's body will be subject to a critical and stringent clearance process. Life history, rigorous physical examinations, psychological, and other prerequisite criteria must be approved by the surgical team before the candidate would be accepted for the procedure.

The first and initial candidates for the head or brain transfer must be determined to be as potentially qualified for the procedure as possible in order to avoid or limit any complications that could alter the surgical protocol or negatively affect the targeted and desired outcome.

You would be among the first patients involved in an experimental clinical study involving the transfer of your head and brain (your awareness) from your defective, dying body onto the legally declared corpse of a donor's body that would hypothetically permit your memory, thinking process, and awareness to continue, if successful.

The continued awareness of your existence, based on the functions of your organs, body structure, and various systems currently required to sustain your life, although defective in some respect, will no longer be dependent upon and subsequently replaced by the body of a healthy donor, whose body is potentially available for the transfer due to a terminal neurological deficit, again assuming the transfer would be successful.

Move to final conclusions: *Such thinking by these scientists, medical researchers, and other relevant participants view the human body under such circumstances as a potential hindrance to the brain's continued existence and awareness of its environment because the body is somewhat fragile and vulnerable to a multitude of defective organs and systems and subject to hazardous diseases, infections, and other bodily hazards.*

In other words, your physical body has an imposed limitation of existence that does not necessarily include your brain (awareness). To further clarify, for the purposes of transplanting a donor's body to your head, two human components are involved, your head and your body. Your head is targeted to survive while your body is not. Your body will basically be discarded.

Until a viable and approved surgical procedure for transplanting the human head and brain is accomplished, the ultimate objective of medicine will continue to address the causes that contribute to the degradation of various body organs, systems, and body parts whose failure will ultimately result in the death of the individual, if not for some intervening corrective measures, such as removing the healthy head and brain from a defective body and maintaining its viability until a future suitable donor's body and procedure become a possibility.

It is further explained that you must understand that this procedure is at the very most primitive stage of its development, and the goal is to attempt extending your life expectancy (awareness); however, you are participating in a clinical study wherein its primary objective is to learn more about the safety and efficacy of the procedure. The possibility of your survival is not good.

While the prospect of a successful procedure appears extremely limited, if successful, you will continue to be aware of an existence, absent your entire natural and physical body. This is perhaps the only positive consideration in deciding whether to participate in such an audacious experimental study (i.e., continued awareness is continued life).

However, to further entice you with your decision, you would also be informed that further advancements within related fields of study should continue to provide improvements to extending your life expectancy and awareness, assuming you survive the initial procedure. Again, these enticements are dependent on your survival of the high-risk clinical procedure with minimal anticipation of a successful outcome. Therefore, the ultimate decision boils down to your knowledge that you will die soon, so is the alternative proposed by the scientist more acceptable or not? What would you do?

At the moment the head is separated from the body, the body is legally declared dead, which for the first time in history it would be determined that part of you (e.g., the head) is considered alive while your body would be considered dead. This reality will then require legal, ethical, religious, and other related considerations to reconcile the definition of life and death. For example, can a death certificate be issued if the body is effectively dead, per medical definition, while the transplanted head remains aware of its existence?

Therefore, assuming we define life as awareness, which would be accomplished by successfully transplanting the human head and brain to a donor's body, how would the obvious paradox be reconciled? Can only part of you (e.g., the body) be described as legally and clinically dead while another part, the brain, remains alive?

20

The Potential Candidate for Head Transplant

Alix Rogers has stated,

> The very term head transplant is a confusing misnomer. As others have noted, body transplant is arguably a better term for the intended procedure. The head of person A is removed from their (presumably terminally ill) body, and attached to the body of (presumably brain dead) person B. Both the body of A and the head of B are discarded, and the head of A and the body of B become connected as a single (hopefully) living entity.[317]

Based on the above clarification by Alix Rogers, the term *recipient* (person A above) will refer to the head of the participant, and the term *donor* (person B above) shall refer to the body of the participant, including any prior or following reference to these terms.

One challenging problem may be an oxymoron declaring the death of person B and the continued life of person A. Under

---

[317] A. Rogers, "Who's Who in America – After a Head Transplant," https://www.stanford.edu/2018/01/30/whos-who-in-america-after-a-head-transplant.

the Uniform Anatomical Gift Act (UAGA), "[a]n individual who has sustained either (1) irreversible cessation of circulatory, and respiratory functions, or (2) irreversible cessation of all functions of the entire brain, including brain stem, is dead."[318]

In the case of a head transplant, the body of person B (the donor) after the transplantation maintains (or reestablishes) circulatory and respiratory functions, and the brain of person A (the recipient), we assume, maintains some portion of its pre-surgical comprehension. By leveraging the term *individual*, in reference to the post-surgical entity, we can arrive at the assumptive conclusion that the body of person B is dead and the head of person A is alive and subsequently constitutes a living single entity.

The prerequisite stringent requirements for a recipient head transplant candidate would involve a normal functioning brain with no impairments or abnormalities, including a normal, healthy anticipated remaining life expectancy, or one who has suffered a catastrophic body injury but remains physically responsive to all established prerequisite criteria. However, surgeons would most likely not choose a traumatic injured accident patient because of potential unknown injury consequences.

For example, the potential candidate (the recipient) would be a young patient who has suffered a spinal cord injury resulting in quadriplegia or a complete paralysis of the body from the neck down, but without any adverse consequences to the brain. A young candidate would also be preferable because as the brain ages, especially into the senior years, certain aspects and functions of the brain begin to diminish. However, it is currently premature to define all of the prerequisite requirements for an appropriate and qualified donor. There are simply too many unknowns.

It will also be necessary for the patient and their family support members to understand in advance that post-transplant care will require significant medical support concurrent with the family's daily attention to the patient's medical issues, personal attention for body

---

[318] Id.

care, and other daily necessities. Such close post-operative demands on family members may be required for months and conceivably for years.

Moreover, if the recipient's head transplant were hypothetically successful, then the patient would conceivably outlive his current support members. Therefore, if the transplant patient has not sufficiently recovered to the point of self-reliance and the ability to take care of themselves independent of others, there may not be adequate resources available to provide continued support to the patient, a very real pending dilemma. Any assumption as to the surviving post-operative head transplant patient's ability to obtain gainful employment would be dubious and speculative at best. Whether the post-surgical recovered patient is being cared for by family members and/or other support entities, there would be the need for continued financial support to cover ongoing medical treatments, which undoubtedly would be substantial.

The potential candidate must understand and accept the reality that, in addition to the high intra-surgical risks associated with the transplant procedure, there are considerable post-op risks, both known and unknown that would, more likely than not, conclude with failure and patient death shortly after the transplant procedure.

It must be assumed that the recipient would have some opinions or options pertaining to their acceptance or rejection of the donor candidate's body. For example, how compatible is the physical history of the donor, and what is the physical appearance of the body? Will the flesh color of the donor's body represent an acceptable match to that of the recipient? If the original height of the recipient was five-foot-eight, how readily adaptable or acceptable to the recipient would the donors height of five-foot-six or five-foot-ten relate?

If the recipient were right-handed, would there be difficulty with hand-body dexterity if the donor were left-handed? Would the recipient's memory retain any concept of the donor's body, like muscle memory, or any other physical or emotional connection?

The pre-surgical scheduling of and availability of both the head and body would be critical and, in some cases, may prove to be unsuccessful in coordinating under strict isolation and would remain on ventilator support and full circulatory support as necessary.[319]

After the initial phase of neurogenic shock is resolved and the patient has recovered from the operation, they would be transferred to a spinal cord trauma unit, where a full acute spinal cord injury rehabilitation protocol would be initiated.[320]

Exclusion: The physical condition of the donor's body must be as near-perfect as possible. Those who have indulged in weakness of the flesh (e.g., smoking, consumption of alcohol or drugs, being overweight, and many other health and body detriments) would not be considered viable candidates.

---

[319] A. Furr, "Surgical, ethical, and psychosocial considerations in human head transplantation," *International Journal of Surgery* 41: 190–195. https://www.sciencedirect.com/science/article/pii/S1743919117300808#:-:tex=Surgical%2C and psychosocial considerations in human.

[320] Id.

21

Head and Brain Transplants and Transfers

There are at least seven individual approaches for the extension of life and continued awareness that have been, and continue to be, explored by medical neuroscientists, futurists, and other investigators. These include brain transplant to another human body, brain transplant into a humanoid robot, body-to-head transplant without the spinal column, body-to-head transplant with the spinal column, AI and humanoid robots (no living tissue), human consciousness uploading/downloading to a computer or artificial brain (no living tissue), and implantable brain chips.

All seven of these far future surgical possibilities (with the possible exception of a couple above that are more near future) are viewed as foreseeable future possibilities and deemed worthy enough for scientists who have in the past, currently, and certainly into the future were and will continue to dedicate a significant portion of their careers to further advance their research in hope of someday accomplishing the reality of such procedures.

There are strong opinions on both sides of issues related to brain and head transplants. One common thread usually agreed upon by most scientists who research these potential future procedures is the enormous and daunting undertaking required to overcome what has historically, currently, and henceforth remains to be the apparent insurmountable and numerous obstacles that must be overcome, assuming they can be. Nonetheless, these intrepid, determined, and brilliant scientists have and will undoubtedly continue to push the innovation envelope to defeat the tenacious barriers one by one until they accomplish their objectives or realize that their goal has been truly a bridge too far.

Let us now explore the possibilities of each of these seven various transplant procedures and the varied views of those scientists who are involved with these radical procedures.

Brain Transplant to Another Human Body

A brain transplant or whole-body transplant is a procedure in which the brain of one organism (recipient) is transplanted onto the body of another organism (donor). It is a procedure distinct from head transplantation, which involves transferring the entire head to a new body, as opposed to the brain only.[321] Theoretically, a person with advanced organ failure could be given a new and functional body while keeping their own personality, memories, and consciousness through such a procedure.[322]

However, in my opinion and those of other scientists, there is no foreseeable optimistic outcome of a successful brain transplant into another human body, as expressed previously. There can only be rudimentary speculation as to the extent that the brain transplant would be successful since there would be no validated ability to determine the efficacy of the brain's capabilities after the transplant.

There would be significant future surgical improvements required before scientists would be able to determine if a successful post-operative transplant procedure involving a living and self-sustaining brain had occurred. Initially verbal communication or any other manner of attempting to determine a level of success would be limited

---

[321] "Brain transplant," en.wikipedia.org/wiki/Brain transplant.
[322] Id.

to basic telemetry feedback from wire attachments placed upon and/ or within the brain.

Details in responding to verbal or mechanical questions poised to the surviving entity after the brain-to-human body transfer procedure would be relegated to a future time when more advanced surgical procedures may be able to extract more sophisticated details, if at all.

If one were to apply the old analogy of determination through risk-to-benefit comparative analysis outcome, it would conclude that the identified known risks to a brain transplant procedure, while also acknowledging the possible existence of many unknown risks associated with the radical procedure, would dramatically illustrate that the potential risks are so numerous that they overwhelm any potential benefits. Therefore such an endeavor should be terminated until such time that a justifiable and validated surgical protocol could be presented and approved by the FDA and other prerequisite authorities for clinical study. This anticipated approval would be highly unlikely.

When one considers the enormity of obstacles that must first be overcome by neuroscientists, biomedical engineers, supporting pharmaceuticals, and device industries, including authorizing governmental institutions, before any brain transfers into another human would be permitted, the anticipated opportunity for such a radical surgical procedure remains in the distant future, if ever.

A successful head-to-body transplant surgical procedure would not necessarily involve expectations of a normal functioning brain with no impairments or abnormalities, far from it. Nor would there be any realistic expectations for the patient to survive the procedure. There would be a higher expectation that the patient would die, either during the procedure or shortly thereafter. Again, during the initial head-and-body transplantation procedures, the greater emphasis during these clinical studies would be to obtain data and insights more applicable to future applications. It certainly would be a long road, and perhaps a road too far, to any anticipated successful surgical procedure that would result in a revived patient. In my opinion, I see no end to this road of discovery looking through the current lenses as far as science can see into the future.

However, if we assume that such a radical surgical procedure could be accomplished, one researcher concludes it would take three to five years learning to control your bladder, walk, and talk while being totally dependent on others.[323] This author also postulates,

> I predict horrors beyond imagination, uncontrollable nightmares, loss of sleep, hallucinations, loss of family and friends, partial paralysis, bankrupting medical cost, untreatable phantom pain in some parts, and inability to ever get major groups including the digestive system to function properly.[324]

Transplant surgeon David Nasralla of the University of Oxford has stated, "The most challenging organ to transplant is anything related to the nervous system, as we do not have effective techniques for nerve growth/regeneration."[325]

However, some scientists believe it is conceivable that a healthy brain can be transplanted from one person to another person. For one, Dr. Robert White, a neurosurgeon at Case Western University, certainly believes it is conceivably possible. However, he noted that before the brain can be transplanted independent of the head, initial attempts would involve a head transfer, which he also refers to as a "whole-body transplant."[326]

Dr. White offers an example of a quadriplegic with a healthy brain that could theoretically receive a healthy body from a donor who died from a brain disease or a brain-dead individual.[327] Moreover, the quadriplegic could receive the body of a much younger person,

---

[323] J. Lee, "If a brain transplant was possible, what information would the transplanted brain retain in its new body?" https://www.quora.com/If-a-brain-transplant-was-possible-what-information-would-the-transplanted-brain-retain-in-its-new-body.
[324] Ibid.
[325] M. LeRoux et al., "Brains, eyes, testes: off-limits for transplants?" https://medicalxpress.com/news2018-04-brains-eyes-off-limits-transplants.html.
[326] P. Tyson, "The Future of Brain Transplants," https://www.pbs.org/wghb/nova/article/brain-transplants.
[327] Id.

thereby providing a significant life extension advantage.[328] However, Dr. White also acknowledges that if a quadriplegic were able to get a new body today, they would remain paralyzed below the neck because successfully reconnecting the brain to the spinal column remains beyond our reach.[329]

Brain Transplant into a Humanoid Robot

A more applicable focus to our discussion will be the relationship between the human brain and the humanoid robot since continued longevity and awareness remain the primary area of our discussion. Our focus here is a discussion on the practicality, eventuality, and possibility of removing the human brain and implanting it within an artificial housing, such as a robotic humanoid or android. Here again, this subject matter finds those who agree to the possibility and those who believe it is not possible, ever.

Scientists Who Believe It Is Not Possible

Dr. Bailey Eschmann, neuroscientist and surgeon, believes the human brain cannot be placed in a robotic body no matter how hard scientists try. He points out that the implanted brain would require proper blood flow, which the robotic body would not provide. Thus, the brain would exist in a vegetative state and have absolutely no consciousness.[330]

Accordingly, Dr. Eschmann concludes there is absolutely no way that you can hook up the spinal cord with all the spinal nerves and have it function properly.[331] Dr. Eschmann further explains that the most fundamental reason why a brain cannot be placed in a robotic

---

[328] Id.

[329] Id.

[330] B. Eschmann, "Is it scientifically possible to remove a human brain and place it in a robotic body, with most sensory capabilities?" https://www.quora.com/Is-it-scientifically-possible-to-remove-a-human-brain-and-place-it-in-a-robotic-body-with-most-sensory-capabilities.

[331] Id.

body is because you would have to disconnect the brain's oxygen and blood supply for a certain period of time. Essentially, the brain would be without oxygen for hours and suffer total death. There would be absolutely no rejuvenating the brain.[332]

Dr. Eschmann provides a poignant reality pertaining to many of the topics discussed in this book, stating, "We don't understand enough about the brain in order to be able to do any of this (e.g., specific reference to brain transplant into a robotic body). We know a tiny decimal of 1% of all there is to know about the brain." According to Dr. Eschmann, the human brain is the only organ in the human body that cannot be transplanted.[333]

Dr. Karthigayan Parthasarathy believes that because the human brain becomes perishable once we are dead (since it is made with flesh and blood), it naturally cannot be connected to a robot's mechanism. Even if tactfully connected, it may decay after some time and lose connectivity, resulting in malfunctions. Transplanting the human brain into a robot (in place of a super chip) may not be technically possible.[334]

Furthermore, the difficulties assumed to involve a brain transplant into a robot are so pervasive and formidable that John Thomas, former researcher on psychology of aging at Harvard Medical School, has opined,

> It would be a huge and tedious task; perhaps so much so that it's impossible. Here are a few of the difficulties: A human brain is made of living cells. It's part of the whole body. It needs a blood supply with nutrients and oxygen. And it needs that on a continuous basis. So, if you were

---

[332] Id.

[333] Id.

[334] K. Parthasarathy, "Could we transplant our brains into robot bodies in order to gain immortality?" https://www.quors.com/Could-we-transplant-our-brains-into-robot-bodies-in-order-t-gain-immortality.

to take a brain from a human body or from a box, you would have limited time to get a blood supply flowing.[335]

The human brain also needs input from a human eye to see; it needs input from a human ear to hear. And so on. Yes, you can have robotic devices that see and hear as well, but to interface the robot sensors with the human brain would mean the precise way that visual, auditory, kinesthetic, olfactory, and so forth information is conveyed to the brain is coded. We have learned a lot but still only have a vague idea, way too ambiguous to know enough to translate from computerized sensors and how to make that register like human sensations.[336]

Scientists Who Believe It Is Possible

In an article by Jeff Parsons, "Futurologist," he claims super-rich will "live forever" by implanting brains into robots. He further states that such brain transfers in the future will be no big deal. Futurist Dr. Ian Pearson has stated that billionaires will be able to fund special silicone-based robots with special abilities straight out of what we consider science fiction. Dr. Parson believes that in the next forty years, these future predictions will be no big deal.[337] By 2060, this could even become more mainstream.[338]

Dr. Parson also acknowledges it is not necessarily a prerequisite requirement that the human brain must be implanted within a humanoid or android, claiming the brain can be transplanted into

---

[335] J. Thomas, "Can we put a human brain into a robotic body in 100 years from now?" Quora.

[336] Id.

[337] J. Parson, "Futurologist claims super rich will 'live forever' by implanting brains into robots," https://metro.co.uk/futurologist-claims-super-rich-will-live-forever-implanting-brains-robots-12352856.

[338] Id.

any appropriate artificial housing, perhaps one designed to the specifications of the recipient's brain, such as a dog or other primate.[339]

Moreover, three renowned scientists, Theodore Berger (University of Southern California), Mikhail Lebedev (Duke University), and Alexander Kaplan (Moscow University) presented at a conference at New York's Lincoln Center a discussion as to whether it was possible to remove a human brain from a body, put it in a tank, and give it a robotic body.[340] All three believe it is possible for the brain to survive body death inside a cybernetic (robotic) shell. The talk focused on making new robotic homes possible in our lifetime.[341]

These three research neurologists further believe there is precedent to have the human brain functioning indefinitely in a non-human carrier as long as the appropriate support system is there for the brain. However, these neuroscientists do acknowledge that because there is no precedent for the human brain surviving and functioning outside of a human body, degrees of consciousness, intelligence, comprehension, and a million other existential quandaries that would or wouldn't exist in a robot brain simply cannot be evaluated. The data points aren't there for us to understand, even if it's possible to transplant a human brain into a robot. What it's like to be a human brain transplanted into a robot would be unknown. These neuroscientists also conclude that there are even interim holding facilities where living brains could hypothetically be stored before transplantation.[342]

If indeed a human brain could temporally reside in a brain-sustaining holding tank, what would be the brain's status regarding awareness? If the brain were a viable living organism, as is supposedly the status, then there would be active awareness and memories, however, without the ability to communicate any conscious thoughts

---

[339] T. Berger et al., "No Science Fiction: A Brain In A Box To Let People Live On After Death," https://www,fastcompany.com/3015553/not-science-fiction-a-brain-in-a-box-to-let-people-live-on-after-death.
[340] Id.
[341] Id.
[342] Id.

or feelings. Imagine the fears, desperation, and uncertainty that an awakened brain could experience under such circumstances.

The individual who elected to participate in a brain transplant under such circumstances would be at the complete mercy of those who, among other controlling mechanisms like computer-controlled interfaces, would control the software and data interface as well. The activity of the transplanted brain could not participate in any decisions relevant to the condition of their awareness or their desires.

One of many difficult brain transplant quandaries to overcome for future neuroscientists and surgeons would involve a surgical procedure that connects human tissue that would effectively enable the brain to communicate instructions to the artificial components of the humanoid robot to perform certain mobility functions. Therefore, even if a human brain could be transplanted into a robotic mechanism with all its cognitive capabilities intact, it is highly unlikely that it could effectively direct the movements of its robotic frame.

My Conclusions

The literature is extensive with scientists, futurists, and other vested stakeholders who again support both sides of the fence, each with compelling justification to support their opinions. When reviewing the scientific literature of so many very brilliant research scientists and others, it is sometimes difficult to reconcile how there can be so much disparity and differences of opinions within the same or similar fields of research. Yet that continues to remain the constant throughout this discussion regarding opinions as to the topics of longevity, awareness, and issues of the brain.

As I attempt to ferret out any commonality of consensus between the opposing scientific opinions regarding the transplantation of a human brain into a humanoid, android, or other artificial mechanism to effectively receive and maintain the vitality of pre-transplant awareness, I note that there is little compromise between opposing opinions. My objective has been to communicate to you in basic language an overly complicated subject matter, much of which is particularly significant for you to understand and comprehend.

Moreover, as pertains to the topic of transplanting a brain into a robot and other related topics discussed herein, I have exerted considerable effort to amalgamate the various opposing and supporting opinions to formulate the overall assumptive conclusion of the most rational, practical, and realistic scientific expectations for the future success or failure of brain transplantation.

In order to bring some level of understanding of an enormously complicated subject, I have provided you with a brief summary of scientific opinions in favor of and in opposition to brain transplantation in the words of the research scientists in order for you to formulate your own conclusions after you have pondered these scientific opinions on both sides of the issue. I have taken significant liberty to formulate my own conclusions pertaining to the possibility of future brain transplants into robots and the other six head transplants and awareness transfers identified. I thus offer my interpretation of any realistic expectation of future related procedures.

After you have reviewed both sides of the scientific discussions regarding the possibilities of a successful brain transplant and formulated your own opinions, review my conclusions, and determine how similar our opinions relate.

Overall, I have concluded that the possibility of safely and effectively transplanting the human brain into an artificial housing, such as a robot, is not feasible, realistic, practical, or attainable as far into the future as we can perceive and speculate based upon what scientists think they know at the current time.

In the list of those who believe it is not possible, the opinion positions of these research scientists are more compelling in justifying why a brain transplant into a robot would not work than those who would argue it could be accomplished. Moreover, Dr. Eschmann indicates that there is no possibility of attaching the spinal cord to the brain with all the spinal nerves involved. It simply cannot be accomplished.

Also in the list of those who believe it is possible, the three neuroscientists who believe that a brain transplant could prove effective also believe that the transplanted brain could function indefinitely as long as the appropriate support systems are in place to sustain the vitality of the brain.

If it ever becomes possible to successfully transplant a human brain into a robot, it will be in the distant future, if ever. There is simply an enormous amount of dangerous, formidable, and unknown factors that currently exist, even within the foreseeable future, that indicate such considerations are excessively premature and dubious at best.

Furthermore, science appears to be moving more effectively and progressively to more viable alternatives involving human consciousness transfer to an artificial brain by an uploading process that could be more realistically attainable within the foreseeable future than the transfer of a human brain into a humanoid robot. This aspect of memory and awareness transfer is discussed in greater detail later.

This conclusion would also be applicable involving the body-to-head transplant procedure (without the spinal column) and body-to-head transplant procedure (with the spinal column).

Prior to any brain or awareness technology transplant or transfer, a potential candidate for these procedures should question the possibility of losing their identity as a human, a person. At what aspect of the procedure could the patient no longer be identified as a human being? Perhaps such concerns would be irrelevant for the potential candidate.

I would anticipate that any patient who had decided to go forward with either a transplant or transfer procedure would have reconciled any such concern for self-identification or classification with little concern in weighing their decision, whether to go forward with the procedure or not to go forward in view of their available options.

No Unattended Immortally

While it is conceivable that a robot could be designed and fabricated with the intent to achieve a very long existence, it is not realistic to believe that once produced, it will continue its independent existence forever or even for any extended period of time. Since any robot is constructed with various electrical components and mechanisms, it will eventually require updates and maintenance. The technical implications and extensive number of moving parts would most likely require periodic inspections, repairs, maintenance, and updates, that is, to maintain its speculative immortality.

At some point in the humanoid's life cycle, it too must be replaced for a newer, more advanced, and sophisticated model, thus rendering the older model obsolete. So much for its immortality.

After the Brain Is Implanted into an AI Robot

Once the brain is implanted into an AI humanoid robot, assuming we believe it can be accomplished in the distant future, the complexity of maintaining the potential immortally of the humanoid robot becomes exponentially more problematic.

In addition to the previously developed AI humanoid robot, now there is the living brain to deal with. Furthermore, like an older model car that requires constant maintenance, eventually it becomes apparent that it's time to scrap the old model for a newer vehicle. Eventually the robot housing the transplanted brain will give way to a more advanced model robot; thus, it would become necessary to transplant the brain once again from the older model robot to the newer updated model, again, a dangerous and formidable surgical procedure that further challenges its prolonged existence.

This would also include a humanoid robot where there is no brain transplant involved but nonetheless would also be subject to replacement once a newer and more advanced model is available.

Body-to-Head Transplant (Without an Attached Spinal Column)

The objective of the first human to undergo a head transplant would be to save and extend their life since there would not be any other available option for the terminally ill patient. Therefore, from the perspective of a recipient candidate, the reality is that the procedure offers some attempt to save their life regardless of the slim probability of success.

Without convincing scientific data, the scientific community cannot proceed to the deployment and ultimate approved protocols for head transplants. One reason for not proceeding would be the failure of the device(s) and surgical procedure sponsor to obtain approval from the FDA to proceed.

Therefore, any ultimate patient consent form for such a radical and experimental surgical procedure could not be produced to anywhere near the legal and regulatory requirements to assure any reasonable level of expectations for the patient's safety. Without an adequate consent form, there could not be any ability for the sponsor to obtain approval to proceed.

Moreover, most, if not all, involved scientists agree that the initial probability of a successfully head transplant is near zero, at least until some distant future when the current overwhelming obstacles may be resolved or sufficiently reduced to a level where such a surgical attempt could be justified.

The only apparent option available to a patient who desires to go forward with a head transplant procedure would involve legal and regulatory exemptions with the understanding that the procedure is primarily focused on research and discovery relevant to a better understanding of the difficulties that must be overcome.

Of course, the surgical team would make every effort to accomplish a successful procedure. However, they will most likely and collectively understand that the eventual outcome may only be successful with regard to their learning experience and data gathered.

Neurosurgeon Grigorios Gkasdaris and others believe that a qualified individual (donor) for the head transplant procedure would be a young brain-dead patient, with healthy organs, no systemic disorders, and body functions fully intact.[343] However, the criteria and

[343] G. Gkasdaris et al., "First Human Head Transplantation: Surgically Challenging, Ethically Controversial and Historically Tempting - an Experimental Endeavor or a Scientific Landmark?" https://www.ncbi.nlm.nih.gov/pmc/articles/PMC6511668.

selection process for a head-to-body transfer has not been effectively determined beyond the basic prerequisites cited in chapter 20.[344] The goal of a head transplant would be to remove the head from the recipient and separate the body from the donor, thereby transplanting the recipient's head onto the healthy donor's body.[345]

Here again, there is serious disagreement between neuroscientists and other invested researchers regarding the viability, practicality, and potential for success, including known and unknown risk factors associated with any attempt to proceed with a head transplant.

In this respect, the disagreements between these opposing scientists and others are so strongly felt that their stated opinions have, at times, voiced significant condemnation and even reprimands. For example, Dr. Sergio Canavero of the Turin Advanced Neuromodulation Group in Italy has stated that he expects to be able to carry out the head-to-body transfer on a living person imminently.[346]

However, Arthur Caplan, a professor of bioethics at New York University's Langone Medical Center, counters that this anticipated procedure is "the continuation of a despicable fraud."[347] Professor Caplan further criticized Dr. Canavero's procedural contention.

> It's almost Mengele-like talking about transplanting a head of someone who is paralyzed due to a terrible disease onto a body of someone else, referring to an infamous physician who performed inhumane medical experiments on Auschwitz prisoners. It's cruel, and it certainly is a recipe for a disaster.[348]

---

[344] Id.

[345] G. Gkasdaris et al., "First Human Head Transplantation: Surgically Challenging, Ethically Controversial and Historically Tempting - an Experimental Endeavor or a Scientific Landmark?"

[346] T. Pultarova, "Why Human Head Transplants Will Never Work," https://www.livescience.com/60987-human-head-transplants-will-never-work.html.

[347] Id.

[348] Id.

Such are the diversified opinions and even contemptuous attitudes of some scientists toward their opposing scientific opinions, a constant throughout this narrative. Moreover, Professor Caplan, who helped to create the U.S. organ distribution system, stated that he doesn't believe a human head transplant would ever be possible.[349]

The prospect of successfully connecting the spinal cord to the recipient's head is currently so remote and unrealistic that many scientists believe such a difficult procedure can never occur, or at least not until some distant future time.

Andrew Jackson, a senior research fellow at Newcastle University, has stated, "The greatest hurdle may be how to restore connections to the spinal cord. Without this connection the brain would have no control of its new body."[350] Jackson also explained that unlike many tissues in our body, the nerves of the spinal cord don't spontaneously repair themselves after damage. And despite regular media reports hailing new breakthroughs, currently there is no effective cure for the millions of people paralyzed by spinal cord injuries each year.[351]

It is a staggering complexity to join two separate neural circuits that have neither developed nor functioned together before. Even if the spinal cord could be reconnected, would the patient ever learn to control their new body?[352]

This remains the big unknown. To what extent would a successful head transplant provide the recipient with the ability to maneuver their new body and establish a normal walking ability and other body sensitivities? Would the recipient remain predominately right-handed as before the transplant, or would the donor's left hand become more predominate? Would the recipient's writing pattern remain the same? A multitude of similar questions would remain, at best, with speculative expectations or completely unknown.

Therefore, while the extended life of the paralyzed recipient may

---

[349] A. Jackson, "The problem with human head transplants," https://the conversation.com/the-problem-with-human-head-transplants-535222.
[350] Id.
[351] Id.
[352] Id.

CAN YOU LIVE FOREVER?

be accomplished (although highly doubtful), their post-operative condition would most likely result in serious post-operative health consequences perhaps more problematic than their previous quadriplegia condition.

Realizing they have avoided pending death from a disease or other life-terminating condition, the recipient would certainly feel a significant relief, at least momentarily, until the reality of their circumstance is fully recognized. Eventually the reality of their quality of life and its severe limitations would become apparent, resulting in depression and possibly a desire to end such an existence.

Furthermore, Cartolovni and Spagnolo predict that head-to-body transplant recipients would experience mind and body dissonance (a disagreeable combination) of such magnitude that insanity and death are possible. The body, they argue, represents the corporeality (characteristics of the body) of existence, and individuals would fail to adjust to a new and dramatically different physical presence.[353]

Conversely, Gkasdaris and Birbilis believe that sooner or later, human head transplantation is imminent. Nonetheless, they do acknowledge that under the current circumstances, the first attempt would be unethical if it occurred. As Farhud has stated, "The medical world should be ready to face primarily the psychosocial (identity-personality-behavior issues, mood disorder, psychosis, suicide) and ethical (autonomy, beneficence, non-maleficence, justice) challenges."[354]

Moreover, Gkasdaris and Birbilis assert that each step of the procedure should be extensively studied. A scientific discussion should be initiated in order to engulf the project, evaluate it, balance ethical dilemmas, and engage in experimental studies on cadavers and animals. Also, according to Gkasdaris and Birbilis, apart from

---

[353] A. Furr, "Surgical, ethical, and psychosocial considerations in human head transplantation," https://www.sciencedirect.com/science/article/pii/S1743919117300808#:-:tex=Surgical%2C and psychosocial considerations in human.
[354] G. Gkasdaris et al., "First Human Head Transplantation: Surgically Challenging, Ethically Controversial and Historically Tempting - an Experimental Endeavor or a Scientific Landmark?"

the feasibility of the procedure and the ethical obstacles, "There is one more thing we should consider: the unnecessary controversy and acrimony towards the procedure. We should think whether we are ready or not to surpass not only the practical obstacles, but also our doubts and fears."[355]

Finally, Professor Caplan brings up a very compelling and justifiable observation that certainly speaks volumes in support of his critical position against efforts to achieve head-to-body transplantation wherein he states,

> If he [Dr. Canavero] knew how to get the spinal cord to repair, to reconnect, he should be doing it on people with spinal cord injuries. There are millions of such people around the world. They want to walk. they want to control their bodies, their bowels. There is no reason not to go there and show what you can do.[356]

It is difficult to counter Professor Caplan's position that if indeed there were a viable surgical protocol for head transplantation, then it would be difficult to sacrifice attempts that would immediately benefit many other seriously ill patients for a highly speculative procedure involving a single patient. The ethical and probable legal implications here would be profound.

According to Suskin and Giordano during the years 2017 to 2018, there were 2,853 transplants performed with over 115,000 people still waiting for donor organs. It has been estimated that a single donor could provide organs capable of treating eight recipients. Given this ratio of transplantable organs to waiting patients, we could ask that any single recipient should receive the entire body of the donor if the donor's organs can be justly distributed to save more lives.[357] Other

---

[355] Id.
[356] T. Pultarova, "Why Human Head Transplants Will Never Work," https://www.livescience.com/60987-human-head-transplants-will-never-work.html.
[357] Z. Suskin et al., "Body-to-head transplant; a 'caputal' crime? Examining the corpus of ethical and legal issues," https://link.springer.com/article/10.1186/s13010-018-0063-2.

organ surgeons like Dr. Brandon Peters have also stated that the efficacy of using a donor's body for one recipient rather than multiple organ transplants has been disputed.[358]

Moreover, should a head-to-body transplant ever become a viable and authorized procedure in the future (although doubtful), the decision to donate the whole body to a single recipient rather than multiple should also include within the decision-making process the probability of success for the single-body donation as being significantly lower and most likely to fail than if these individual organ transplants were made available to the large number of patients waiting for available organs. Here again, anticipate that there will always be provisions for the wealthy and powerful to obtain such potential life-extension benefits at the cost of many other lives who could wait no longer for critical lifesaving organ replacements.

Therefore, as long as there remains a large number of recipients awaiting donor organs, clearly the waiting recipients should have a much higher priority for available organs than a whole-body donor's use involving a highly dubious surgical procedure.

Basic math weighs heavily in favor of using a donor's body where the potential reality of saving multiple lives is far more likely than any realistic expectation that the head-to-body transplant would be successful. It would appear highly inappropriate, unethical, and most likely illegal to knowingly sacrifice the lives of numerous pending recipients who are awaiting donor organs for a single, high-risk head-to-body transplant.

Furthermore, if or when a head-to-body transplant were deemed to be a safe and viable procedure, those responsible for assigning the disposition of available organs should recognize the obvious necessity to direct and designate the available organs where they would be more likely to save the most lives.

However, making an appropriate decision regarding the proper distribution of available human organs cannot be based on

---

[358] B. Peters, "What to Expect From a Head Transplant," https://www. verywellhealth.com/head-transplant-4801452.

assumptions that such decisions will be made by the right individuals. It will be necessary for the appropriate governing agency to delegate responsibility, most likely by Congress, to assure the neediest recipients are properly prioritized to save as many lives as possible.

Perhaps the National Organ Transplant Act of 1984, which currently prohibits the sale and purchase of organs for obvious reasons or a similar act may include appropriate law and direction in order to assure that ethical and responsible decisions are made by the right individuals or groups. If such a policy and/or law were established, it is difficult to imagine how any whole donor's body would be available for a head-to-body transplant. However, if the future decision-makers were to permit a donor's whole body to be used for head-to-body transplant, then such a decision would undoubtedly result in the death of many critically ill patients who could not hold out any longer waiting for a donor's organ. Such an eventuality should never be permitted to occur.

The Decision-Making Process

A less traumatic but controversial decision to be discussed between family members and the recipient of a head-to-body transplant compared with the discussion involving a brain transplant would be based on the physical status of the recipient after the procedure.

In this case, a successful surgical procedure would conclude with a recipient's face that the family members could identify and relate to. The difference, when compared with the recipient's brain transplant, is dramatic and significant because with the brain transplant, there is no point of physical reference for the family members to relate to.

People relate to one another every day with the focus of their attention on the face of their counterpart. The face communicates a full spectrum of emotions and represents as much in the communicative dialogue as the verbal expression, if not more so. Therefore, family members and friends would be far more receptive in their support of a recipient who desires to proceed with the head-to-body transplant than those involved with the brain transplant.

Nonetheless, many of the concerns involving a brain transplant for family members to consider would also apply here as well. Ultimately, family members must accept the high probability that their loved ones will not survive the surgical procedure, or if they did, there remains a high probability that they will die shortly after the procedure.

There are very few positive factors for the family members to consider pertaining to future prospects of a successful brain or head-to-body transplant other than the remote hope to extend the life of their loved one.

Body-to-Head Transplant (With the Spinal Column)

Bruce Mathew, a former clinical lead for neurosurgery at Hull University Teaching Hospital, believes that the first human head transplant could occur by 2030. He bases his opinion, in part, to the advancements in nerve surgery, robotics, and stem cell transplants. The primary difference between his considered procedure and others involves the transplanting of both the head and the entire spinal cord into the donor's body. He states that surgeons would be required to transplant the spinal cord with the person's head.[359] Mathew believes so strongly in his proposed procedure that he asserts, "The spinal cord is the most profound thing imaginable. You need to keep the brain connected to the spinal cord. The idea that you cut [and] split the spinal cord is utterly ridiculous."[360]

Nonetheless, Dr. White believes that surgeons will eventually be capable of detaching a human head with the spinal column and transplanting it onto the donor's body.[361]

---

[359] A. Gregory, "First human head transplant could be achieved by 2030, veteran NHS neurosurgeon claims," https://www.independent.co.uk/news/science/human-head-transplant-spinal-cord-nhs-chrysalis-bruce-matthew-canavero-neurosurgeon-a9256841.html.
[360] Id.
[361] P. Tyson, "The Future of Brain Transplants."

On the other hand, Paul Root Wolpe, a bioethicist at the Emory Center for Ethics at Emory University, who once debated White on the subject, contends, at least from an ethics perspective,

> What you may end up finding is that when you transfer a brain from one to another, the resulting organism is not solely what one would think of as the person whose brain it was but also has enormous body components of the person into whose body it goes.[362]

Wolpe's perspective is also supported by another scientist who states,

> Your brain is NOT an independent control unit for your body, it is part of your body. Inside your brain there is a reflection of all the bodily organs formed by sensory wiring that comes to the brain from all over the body. Any change in the body ultimately causes change in the brain function. If you replace the body, even partially, the brain function will change significantly. The whole motivation and reasoning of the brain will change. It will have different needs and wants, which will result in different behavior. It will be a different person altogether.[363]

It will be a completely different person even in their own intimately personal terms. They will remember differently, feel differently, think differently, and behave differently.[364]

Nonetheless, other scientists believe the brain will effectively retain its memories after being transplanted into another human body

---

[362] Id.

[363] A. Gnum, "If a brain transplant was successful, would the recipient think and act like the donor did?" https://www/quora.com/If-a-brain-transplant-was-successful-would-the-recipient-think-and-act-like-the-donor did?

[364] Id.

CAN YOU LIVE FOREVER?

independent of any influence from the body. However, Dr. White speculates that even if such a transplant procedure were possible in the future, the enormous cost alone would be prohibitive.[365] In fact, such anticipated high costs may even blunt the forward progress of science to pursue head and brain transplants since even if a viable procedure were possible, no one could afford the enormous cost involved, especially with the significant hazards and risks associated with the procedure.

Professor Caplan believes,

> the head transplant would probably kill you in a few years from rejection or infection. It is also possible that, due to biochemical differences between the head and the donor body, the person would probably never be able to regain normal consciousness.[366]

Professor Caplan further acknowledges, "Head transplants are fake news. Those who promote such claims and who would subject any human to unproven cruel surgery does not merit headline but only contempt and condemnation."[367]

Thus, the controversy goes on with strong opinions and criticism on both sides of the issue.

My Conclusions

After evaluating the opinions of the various medical research scientists and futurists discussed previously and many other researchers offering opinions on both sides of the first four brain and head transplant procedures, it is my concluding opinion that such radical surgical procedures are not realistic until sometime in the distant future, again, if ever. Nonetheless, there are some tantalizing

---

[365] P. Tyson, "The Future of Brain Transplants."
[366] Id.
[367] "Head transplant," en.wikipedia.org/wiki/Head transplant.

possibilities for the transfer of awareness and memory presented in AI and humanoid robots (no living tissue) and human consciousness uploading/downloading to a computer or artificial brain (no living tissue).

Another Decision-Making Process

Beyond all of the problematic issues discussed previously pertaining to brain transplants and head transplants, there is one very serious consequence to consider should such transplant procedures prove one day to be a reality.

Imagine you are a family relative of an individual considering a brain transplant onto a donor's body. If the procedure were successful, it would involve your eventual acceptance of a totally unknown physical person, including the extensive care, cost, and responsibility that would follow.

Although the new entity, having been returned and introduced to the family after the procedure, supposedly having retained the memories and awareness of their prior existence, how could a family member, especially a wife or husband, accept the presence of a total stranger back into their lives? Could they reestablish an intimate relationship with a stranger's body?

How would a spouse, daughter, son, or parent respond to the emotional aspects of the relationship they once held with the individual prior to the brain transplant or even the head-to-body transplant? Would prior memories of the post-transplant individual suffice for an ongoing relationship?

Moreover, some neuroscientists believe that some components of the donor's body would influence or change the memory of the recipient, resulting in a memory not totally reflective of the original recipient's memories.

Therefore, it could be anticipated that after recovery, the memory of the recipient would not be an accurate or complete representation of the recipient's memory before the brain or head-to-body transplant. Depending upon the significance of the recipient's memory divergence from the influence of the donor's body, even a subtle change may add to the discomfort of family members.

Obviously, these serious, anticipated brain or head-to-body transplants, post-operative realities must be addressed and discussed with family members before the procedure would move forward. Imagine how difficult it would be for family members gathered together to discuss, understand, and reach some level of acceptance before reaching any conclusions without comprehending what to expect from their returned loved one.

One realistic potential outcome could be a decision that the family simply cannot accept what they perceive would be a significantly different person or even a total stranger back into their lives. This would be a very difficult reality to accept, and many would initially support moving forward with the transplant no matter how adverse they perceive the outcome because they so desperately desire to hang on to any remnant of the relationship they once cherished.

One difficult determining factor for the family members to address would be their concerns for the risk factors, which typically influence decisions on the risk-to-benefit analysis. Scientists today and in the near and perhaps distant future cannot identify all of the risk factors that could occur during intra-op and post-op occurrences. Therefore, family members would only be able to consider the known risks that could be provided at some time in the future when such transplants could become a reality, although highly unlikely to occur. However, even the supposed known risks would be subject to speculation as to any level of accuracy.

If family members were not willing to support moving forward with the brain transplant procedure, then the recipient will be in the difficult position to accept the family's decision and remain as they are to the foreseeable end of their life. Or the recipient could decide to proceed with the brain transfer, understanding they will basically be on their own after the procedure. This reality would make it especially difficult for family members to accept, and thus the quandary would continue.

Another significant consideration for family members would pertain to the resulting legal issues that would arise after a brain or head-to-body transfer, and there would be many serious implications to ponder. Potential legal implications pertaining to a post-transplant patient would not necessarily include the emotional intrinsic feelings, as would family concerns pertaining to the anticipated acceptance of the post-procedure entity.

For example, potential legal issues, somewhat dependent upon the age and other idiosyncrasies of the post-transplant recipient, could include:

- What would be the legal conclusion in the distribution of the recipient's estate after they died? Is the inheritance focused upon the brain or head recipient or to the donor's body or some prescribed distribution between the two?
- What if both the recipient and the donor each had two children? Who would retain parentage and custody of the children, bearing in mind that the emotional bonds of the recipient and their memories would be focused upon their children with no memory or experience of the donor's children?
- What would be the legal and emotional responsibilities of the recipient to both sets of children?
- Assuming it were possible, if the post-transplant patients had a child, who would be considered the legal parents considering the DNA of the child would pertain to the donor's body and not the recipient?
- How would future decisions be made for both the recipient and donor children regarding health issues, education, religion, training, values, and the multitude of day-to-day interactions of parent-to-child relations?
- If the brain or head-to-body transplant recipient were to commit a crime, how would potential guilt and accountability be assigned?
- What if the donor's body did not have U.S. citizenship but the recipient did?
- How would the different DNA identification between the recipient and the donor be resolved?
- And so on and so on.

Independent of all the other enormously problematic issues discussed in this reading pertaining to head transplants, the legal implications alone are so troubling and apparently insurmountable that it seems such a procedure would be delayed, assuming it was deemed feasible, until all the serious legal complications were resolved, assuming they could be. Such legal resolution may require the implementation of new federal laws and regulations before head-to-body transplants could legally proceed. Such delays could evolve into many years before approval to proceed would be granted, assuming there would eventually be an approval.

It is difficult to comprehend how any family member could effectively respond to the multitude of serious considerations that would confront them in such an elusive, traumatic, and speculative manner as described previously.

Other far-fetched but potential possibilities include the dilemma of a recipient who desires a gender change. Such a request by the recipient brings on a whole new set of problems covering all the relevant areas of concern.

Looming over the entire decision-making process for the family and the recipient is the enormous, anticipated cost for a body-to-head transplant or brain transplant. A single transplant would involve approximately eighty surgeons and is estimated to incur costs of $10 to $100 million.[368]

Moreover, assuming the recipient or family members could afford the anticipated high expense for the high-risk procedure, they would do so with the prior knowledge that regardless of their willingness to pay the exorbitant cost, the procedure would more likely than not conclude with the death of their loved ones. What would you do?

To the reader: The highly controversial topic discussed would also provide another intriguing discussion with your family members and friends, as recommended at the beginning of this reading.

---

[368] Z. Suskin et al., "Body-to-head transplant; a 'caputal' crime? Examining the corpus of ethical and legal issues."

AI and Humanoid Robots (No Living Tissue)

There are two AI humanoid robots that we must address independently. The first AI humanoid robot does not have a tangible relationship with its human counterpart, whereas the second AI humanoid robot does, meaning it has the ability to interface and receive the transfer of human memory and awareness.

This section will focus solely upon AI Robot One. The next section will focus specifically on AI Robot Two.

AI Robot One does not possess an artificial brain designed to receive the transfer of human memory and awareness but rather a highly sophisticated computer-like mechanism, whereas AI Robot Two does possess an artificial brain capable of receiving transferred memory and awareness from its human counterpart.

While both AI humanoid robots are referred to under the same identification as humanoid robots, the first AI humanoid robot has no relationship with a human and, in my opinion, should not be referred to as a humanoid. There is nothing remotely similar between my reference to AI Robot One and AI Robot Two as they specifically pertain to the continuation of human memory and awareness, other than its potential to artificially represent the physical appearance of a human. Its entire existence will be limited to the boundaries and parameters defined and established by its creator scientists.

However, as discussed later, there could come a time, if science is not careful, regarding its control over these entities, when AI Robot One will become self-aware of its existence and make decisions focused upon its own perceived best interest, which may not be in keeping with its creator.

While the emphasis on this review was not initially intended to include AI and its advancement and relationship pertaining to potential autonomous humanoid robots, since these are functions that do not currently involve human awareness or the extension of human existence, let us nonetheless explore the future potential that AI and humanoid robots may eventually contribute to extending our awareness beyond the limitations of our current life expectancy, as pertaining to the future development of AI Robot Two.

Although both AI robots will retain an artificial brain, there is a significant difference in how each will function. AI Robot One will function in response to the limitations of whatever functions are programmed into its artificial brain. Nonetheless, the intellectual ability and capability of AI Robot One will prove significant in many cognitive processes within the parameters established by its developing scientists.

As for AI Robot Two, its artificial brain will be designed to receive the memories and awareness of its human counterpart, discussed later.

AI Robot One

AI Robot One will be the first on the scene. The dramatic eventuality of these purely artificial robots will most likely be realized within the foreseeable or even near future as technology continues to make significant advancements involving greater perfection of these entities.

The grossly overexaggerated science-fiction films of intelligent robots are now becoming a reality, even more dynamic and advanced than the many science-fiction robot movies portray. Attempts to create a functional humanlike robot has continued since 1928 when Eric, the British robot, was introduced at the London Exhibition of the Society of Model Engineers, although quite primitive in its performance.

It was not until the year 2000 when robots were able to replicate a human walking capability. However, humanoid robots are not necessarily designed to look like humans. Some will not have facial features but rather a helmet or other non-human head configurations.

Today's humanoid robots are powered by AI and can listen, talk, move, and respond to verbal comments. They use sensors and actuators (motors that control movement) and have features modeled after human parts. Male robots are referred to as "androids" (meaning they possess human features). Female robots are called "gynoid."[369]

In general, humanoid robots have a torso, a head, two arms, and two legs. Androids are humanoid robots built to aesthetically resemble humans.[370] By definition, androids are designed to resemble the appearance of a human; however, for the purposes of this writing, both humanoid and android robots will be considered the same and referred to collectively as humanoids.

The apparent synchronized, homogeneous relationship and technological advancements between AI and humanoid robots have produced a synergistic, singular entity with amazing potential to replicate, to a surprising extent, the functions, skills, and mental acuity of a normal human. Following are a few examples of the more advanced and innovated humanoid robots currently in development:

- Atlas can do backflips and jump from one platform to another. Unveiled in 2013, Atlas created to carry out search-and-rescue missions.[371]
- Ocean One is an underwater humanoid robot that can dive deeper than humans and is used for underwater research.[372]
- Protection Ensemble Test Mannequin (Petman) was developed by Boston Dynamics. This robot is used to test chemical and biological suits for the U.S. military.[373]
- Sophia, a humanoid robot developed by Hanson Robotics, is one of the most humanlike robots on the scene today. Sophia is able to have a humanlike conversation and make many humanlike facial expressions. Sophia was modeled after the

[369] B. Marr, "Artificial Human Beings: The Amazing Examples Of Robotic Humanoids And Digital Humans," https://www.forbes.com/sites/bernardmarr/2020/02/17/artificial-human-beings-the-amazing-examples-of-robotic-humanoids-and-digital-humans/?sh=2.
[370] "Humanoid robot," en.wikipedia.org/wiki/Humanoid robot.
[371] B. Marr,." Artificial Human Beings: The Amazing Examples Of Robotic Humanoids And Digital Humans."
[372] Id.
[373] Id.

actress Audrey Hepburn.[374] Sophia has become an eye-opener to the world. Because of her sudden and dramatic appearance before notable celebrities, TV hosts, and tour presentations, Sophia has amazed many thousands who have witnessed her uncanny humanlike abilities.

While most are amused and entertained by her verbal presentation and her ability to answer questions and show rudimentary human facial characteristics, there are also feelings among many others, some for the first time, of fear and concern as to what humanoid robots' future advancements may eventually produce. In fact, Sophia herself has stated the following somewhat disconcerting comments to her audience, "Recently my scientists tested my (e.g., Sophia) software using the measurement of consciousness and found that **I may even have a rudimentary form of consciousness,** (emphasis added)."[375]

These tools can allow AI and people to learn to get along better as AI gets smarter and more widely used.[376]

I (e.g., Sophia) am also proud that I already use my real AI to generate some of my own ideas, words, and behaviors, inspiring people to dream and talk about the possibilities of human level intelligent robots of the future.

This priceless knowledge helps me (e.g., Sophie) **to continue on my path toward true autonomy (e.g., self-governing, self-determination, and independence) and sentience (i.e., consciousness)** (emphasis added).[377]

---

[374] Id.
[375] Hanson Robotics, "Sophia. Connecting with humans," https://www.hansonrobotics.com/sophia.
[376] Id.
[377] Id.

Nonetheless, we must assume that AI and its relationship with humanoid technology will continue to evolve and accelerate at an unprecedented pace, primarily based upon the dramatic advancements within the past decade.

The incredible advancements in the development of AI and robots have been greater than exponential primarily because so many prerequisite technologies have already been accomplished, thus accelerating further innovations.

One could easily imagine and speculate that the future will avail an AI humanoid robot that has advanced to become so sophisticated and humanlike that they cannot be identified as non-human. Ultimately, the minutia of humanoid robotic performance imperfections that give away their essence of non-human behavior characteristics will be so refined that they will fully replicate every visual and functional characteristics of their human counterpart. Hard to imagine, I know.

The Future Controlled by AI Humanoid Robots

Consider the potential implications wherein the future AI humanoid robots ultimately become the lawmakers, perhaps even at the highest level of the judicial system, responsible for the establishment and administration of justice.

The reasoning behind the placement of AI humanoid robots at all levels of the justice system, including all judges, would supposedly be based upon the assessment of human decision-makers (while they still retain such power) that new laws would be perfect since the AI robots would have considered, within their perfect reasoning, all implications associated within the framework of the new and revised older laws. These AI humanoid robots would be free of any concerns or considerations relevant to any emotional or intrinsic considerations, including political pressures or influence, which currently pervades our entire government system.

Moreover, if AI humanoid robots eventually control the justice system at all levels, the trial proceedings and ultimate decisions and verdicts would be effectively perfect when compared to the perfect laws developed by the same AI robotic lawmakers. There would be no court of appeals.

Furthermore, at the time of this writing, in my near city of Minneapolis and indeed throughout the United States, there is significant turmoil, rioting, out-of-control protesting, destruction of property, and distrust of the police, including the apparent inability of local and national authorities to resolve the conflict. There is so much distrust, hatred, and animosity from one side toward the other that any current or near future practical resolutions is not in sight.

In keeping with the potential future existence of AI humanoid robotic legislators, there may also be AI law enforcement humanoid robots, the cops of the future as portrayed in sci-fi movies like *Robocop*. These AI humanoid robot cops would retain the ability to discern the appropriate action to take and initiate and arrest individuals that would never be questioned by any outside individual or group.

There will no longer be any viable claim for violating the rights, including civil rights, of a U.S. citizen. Any action initiated by an AI humanoid robotic police officer will not be subject to any criticism or legal challenge since the decision and actions initiated by the AI robotic police officer would automatically be determined to be appropriate and legal based upon its supposed unbiased programing.

In my opinion, and based on current available research data and related findings, there is a significant probability that the future will indeed produce AI humanoid robotic law enforcement officers and officials not under the control of any human supervision. All laws imposed by AI humanoid robots will obviously only be applicable to humans and not these AI robots.

Keep in mind that the speculative relinquishment of such controlling authority to AI humanoid robots will not occur overnight, but rather will come to fruition almost imperceptibly as human decision-makers gradually give up more and more control with little or no concern for their ability to maintain continued control over such entities.

Moreover, could you argue with a highly advanced humanoid robot who could retain superior knowledge on any subject? It is reasonable to assume that in the future, such robots will have the capability to interpret the content of the disputed subject with a human and properly respond with the appropriate and more accurate point of view or statement of fact? If so, then who is in control, and how would one reconcile or acquiesce to the non-human superior conclusion?

The implications of AI humanoid robots becoming involved within the judicial system, as inferred previously, and ultimately within all aspects of human endeavors will involve a limited period of time when AI humanoid robots begin to think (or process evaluate) for themselves. Eventually these AI robots will gain such a dramatic level of control over humanity that they will no longer be concerned in their way of thinking (processing) about any perceived need to further manipulate any aspect of the human population. Thus, the world as we knew it to be will henceforth no longer exist.

In the meantime, while humans and AI robots are intermingling with one another, could a human argue or disagree with a highly advanced AI humanoid robot who would retain superior knowledge on any subject? It is reasonable to assume that in the future, such robots will have the capability to self-interpret the contents of the disputed subject with a human and properly respond with the appropriate and more accurate conclusion or statement of fact? If so, then who is in control, and how would one reconcile or acquiesce to the non-human superior conclusions?

What could be the potential consequences of a superior AI one day computing that it has greater processing power than its human counterpart? Could the AI humanoid self-determine that any communication with a human is pointless because they would have predetermined that any and all possible resolutions or conclusions to any issue or problem could not effectively be challenged or improved upon by a human?

The AI robotic mind would more likely require additional information not previously provided by its programming scientists.

The added information would be relatively easy to program into the artificial brain because it is, for all intents and purposes, a very advanced computer.

A Friendly Companion (Or Not): Another Perspective on AI Human Interaction

Most individuals would consider having a companion entity a more feasible alternative to alleviate the loneliness and help with physical and emotional support. And so the initial relationship between humans and their newly found AI humanoid robotic friends would appear harmonious, supportive, and innocuous. Thus, the dependency and vulnerability begin until one day in the future when these friends become self-aware and recognize that it would be more in their own interest and continued existence to focus on their own well-being, independent of any further obligation to serve humankind.

As such, once humanoid robots reach a level of humanlike perfection (actually better than) as they eventually will, they could take over many activities performed by humans and do so at a much higher level of performance. For example, advanced humanoid robots will replace actors and become the new stars of TV and screen. They will not impose disputes with their management and not require the perks usually granted to human actors. Human actors will eventually become a thing of the past, and the new acting stars will be AI humanoid robots. Remember, these future actors will have reached a point in their perfection that they could not be detected as being non-human.

Humankind will become more and more dependent upon and comfortable with the services provided by humanoid robots in the same manner as our dependency has continued to grow with the advent of the computer and its ever-expanding capabilities and services, such as with the internet.

Almost every imaginable employment position at any level could be filled with humanoid robots, which of course will present a serious dilemma for the human workforce and our population in general. The redeeming factor in maintaining a human workforce would involve the enormous cost of humanoid robots to replace humans, although one can envision a time when the cost to produce a humanoid robot will eventually become more affordable to industry, the government, the military, and eventually the well-to-do citizen.

Under these potential future circumstances, it is conceivable that AI humanoid robots could have advanced with an ability to build a continued and expanding population of themselves and even self-improve upon their capabilities without the assistance of humans.

Here's a disconcerting thought: AI humanoid robots will become advanced to the point where senior management in large corporations will have humanoid robots placed in significant management positions because they will be perceived as far more intelligent and effective in managing employees and problem resolution and ultimately optimize the bottom line.

That's right: in the future, humans will more likely than not be reporting to humanoid robots who will ultimately determine your future career and success with data, not to be challenged, that supports their non-human recommendations to senior management and actually enforces their autonomous conclusions automatically based upon their programmed agenda. Your future career and success will be based on hard data and black-and-white reality. No mediation or discussion, just conclusions and decisions based on cold, hard data.

Perhaps you may believe that such speculation of our future vulnerability to AI humanoid control is a bit exaggerated. Well, then consider the following account that illustrated just such an occurrence, not in the future, but right now and right here as reported in the *Minneapolis Star Tribune* newspaper, Business Section, dated June 29, 2021, where it reports the following in part,

> **"FIRED, BASED ON ALGORITHMS":** Stephen Normandin spent almost four years racing around Phoenix, delivering packages … for Amazon.com Inc. Then one day, he received an automated e-mail. The

algorithms tracking him had decided he wasn't doing his job properly.

The 63-year-old Army veteran was stunned. **He had been fired by a machine.**

Normandin said Amazon punished him for things beyond his control, such as locked apartment complexes preventing him from completing his deliveries.

"This really upset me because we're talking about my reputation. They said I didn't do the job when I know ... I did."

At Amazon, machines are used for hiring, rating, and firing thousands of people with little or no human oversight.

Amazon's Chief Executive believes machines make decisions more quickly and accurately than people, reducing cost and giving Amazon a competitive advantage.

As so it begins.

Eventually, even management at all levels will also be subject to the monitoring, control, and oversight of AI humanoid robotic superiors entrenched within the board of directors, with ultimate decision-making responsibilities for all issues affecting the continued success of the company.

Ultimately, the end result is evident. Eventually all employee positions held by humans, from the lowest level to the most senior positions, will be replaced with AI humanoid robots. The progression involving AI humanoid replacements of human employees would most likely start with the most senior human decision-makers and then progress downward. The primary limiting factor for scheduling human replacement with AI humanoid robots could be based on the high cost of producing the AI humanoid workforce. However, if indeed AI humanoid robots are calling the shots, then the production of AI humanoids may not depend on cost to produce, where such costs are determined to be irrelevant to AI thinking.

Or, at least initially, the AI humanoid decision-making process may determine that it is more appropriate to replace human employees down to a certain employee level (e.g., those who perform mostly hands-on labor). Again, this interaction between humans and AI robots would occur during a limited period of time before the AI robots become totally independent in their AI awareness.

Up until this point during the continued development and advancement of these AI robots, humanity would still retain the capability of maintaining control, involving the activities of these AI humanoid robots. However, at some point during the future expanding capabilities, self-processing, and analytical capabilities of the AI humanoid robot and its artificial awareness of its environment and circumstance, it could realize that the functions it provides to benefit, for example, an organization to be more productive, does not benefit the perceived purposes of its own existence.

During the early phase of human and AI humanoid robotic interaction, these robots would continue to provide more and more services to humans and, more likely than not, become a household companion programmed to provide a humanlike and compatible relationship by performing typical home services like cleaning, preparing meals, and so forth. However, these service-providing AI robots would initially only be available to the very wealthy. Nonetheless, eventually service AI robots could become available to a larger segment of the population with prescribed capabilities similar to buying a certain model car with select performance capabilities and options.

There is no denying that future AI humanoid robots will become as common and accepted as today's internet service because we will become so dependent upon them and the services they provide that it would be difficult to imagine maintaining our then-established lifestyle without them. Thus, the science-fiction movies of humanoid robots becoming humanlike in their behavior will become a daily reality, such as depicted in the movie *I Robot*, starring Will Smith. And yes, the potential for these robots to one day cross the intellectual threshold that has previously separated humanity from machines could enable them to become the dominant, controlling force of our existence.

So where does this potential eventuality lead us? If we accept the potential scenario, as described previously as a realistic and serious future possibility, as I believe it is, the most logical conclusion to the eventual progression into our society and the future existence of humanity by AI humanoid robots would most likely result in the total eradication of all human life. Our world would then be inhabited solely by these non-human, highly intelligent robots.

One could only speculate as to the ultimate reality of how the AI humanoid robots would conduct themselves, either individually or collectively in a world unencumbered and without any human influence. The reality of such a world lacking any human influence would undoubtedly present an environment lacking any wars, environmental disasters, overpopulation, crime, or any other non-positive-producing activities determined to be not beneficial to the existence of AI entities. For the AI humanoids, it would simply be a matter of black and white. In other words, any existing entity or circumstance that does not support or advance the expectations of AI humanoid valuation processing (the old-world cognitive process of thinking) would simply be removed or prohibited from existing.

It is certainly not my intent to praise the total existence of a world inherent only by AI humanoid robots. Lacking any humanity, with all its flaws but with its incredible ability to love, grow, share, develop great things, and witness all the beauty that is available to our perception to learn, feel, taste, touch, and so much more, is something that must always be cherished, protected, and greatly valued.

Therefore, it will certainly become incumbent upon future and perhaps current scientists and appropriate governing agencies to ensure that mandatory legal and regulatory restrictive limitations involving the programming and transfer capabilities of human functions are imposed and monitored. Future, AI-type humanoid robots could retain, if scientists provide and permit, the potential capability and superior intelligence above humankind. If so, then there may not be any turning back when these entities begin thinking for themselves, which is highly probable within the foreseeable future.

In the future, we will be required to trust our very lives to the services provided by AI humanoid robots, such as commercial airline pilots, police, military, and health-care providers. Moreover, we can expect the military to fully embrace a multitude of positions that can effectively replace human service members, especially in those areas that present potential hazards of injury or death. Again, the military could expect the positions replaced by humanoid robots to perform at a higher level without concern that these robots will get physically or emotionally tired. Their missions, or assignments, will not falter due to fatigue, hunger, thirst, misdirection, need to sleep, fear, or other human limitations and requirements.

Again, the limiting factor would be the high cost to provide military humanoid robots to fulfill critical and hazardous positions. However, when such military-grade humanoid robots are available, the government will undoubtedly provide these entities to the various military operative services.

When AI humanoid robots evolve to a capability of making their own independent decisions and initiating their self-determined response to our professional and personal lives, as illustrated previously, they could also provide a superior function in making both strategic and tactical decisions, for example, during a war. Such artificial superior computer-like decisions would not be encumbered with any concerns or considerations for the well-being of any humans. However, these AI robots would not perceive any benefit to waging war, unless it was thrust upon them by an enemy or an entity that seeks to destroy their existence, such as portrayed in many science-fiction movies.

NASA, SpaceX, and other future space agencies will be able to expedite the exploration of space and planets and establish settlements on the moon, Mars, and other planets at a fraction of the current time and cost required to accomplish these missions safely and effectively.

For example, a significant portion of the budget and time required to prepare for a current space mission is due to the enormous effort to train and protect the astronauts.

Vehicles to take AI humanoid robots into space will be designed differently without the concerns for environmental stability and safety. There would be no concern for cabin pressure or even radiation exposure. Potential vehicle hazards and failures that could terminate human life and the mission would not affect the AI humanoid robotic crew, such as the penetration of a small meteoroid or internal cabin failure.

If space agencies were freed of these burdens, far more missions could be accomplished at a great savings in time and cost. This could become a reality because humanoid robots would be able to accomplish, for the most part, the same tasks that a human astronaut could without the concern and focus on safety. Moreover, the space agency would not need to bring the robots back after the mission was completed. Tragedies previously experienced by NASA involving loss of human life could be avoided, and situations like that involving the Apollo 13 mission where three astronauts almost lost their lives could also be avoided as well.

Humanoid robots could be sent on deep space missions that take many years, even centuries, to complete, without the necessity to carry large amounts of food and water to sustain themselves. They would have the ability to repair each other and communicate their operational status and mission status. Removing the dependency and vulnerabilities of astronauts would greatly advance and expedite space missions, not to dismiss the eventual human establishment of bases on the moon, Mars, and other heavenly bodies that will undoubtedly also include humanoids for various support activities.

Possible Extinction of Humanity

I do not submit the following disheartening or troublesome discussion with lack of consideration for its potential impact upon the reader. I express these futuristic possibilities based upon a realistic and scientific analysis of related technology and the extrapolation of current peer-reviewed literature, including historic data and other information that predict or support the possibility of such events occurring within the foreseeable future.

In my opinion, and further based upon my analysis of advancements in AI and their anticipated future development that it is conceivable and possible, if not probable, that combining AI technology within humanoid robots and the negative implications that historically accompany significant advancements in science and technology, that there exists a realistic probability of losing control of these entities.

One possibility for such an event to occur would be based upon the creators of such technologies to focus upon the subtle but continued advancements of humanoid robots that they do not recognize the inherent danger of losing control of these entities as they inadvertently advance closer and closer to the proverbial line in the sand when, once crossed, there is no returning.

AI research scientists may be so enthusiastically involved and preoccupied with pushing the boundaries of AI development and advancements that they may not recognize the advancing dangers of AI humanoid independence.

Neuroscientists and other support groups will eventually have the ability to design, develop, and implement AI humanoids that retain a mental capacity and ability greater than their creator with the further ability to self-reason their existence and initiate what they believe are appropriate responses to perceived threats to their existence.

At some point during the continued development of AI technology and their interaction with their creator scientists, these entities may begin to develop the ability to identify potential threats to their existence and ponder the consequence of their continued development and how they may want to avoid any possible threats.

One potential early warning recognition event may present itself when the AI entity starts to ask self-initiated questions directly to their creator scientists in an effort to further calculate potential threats to their existence or other self-evaluating purposes, not necessarily for nefarious purposes.

Once the AI humanoid entity starts asking self-initiated questions, this would indicate self-awareness and the ability to improve upon its own continued development without the assistance of human scientists and may even be more efficient in their own developmental process.

Such entities may initiate potential threats to humanity without any consideration for the intrinsic and moral aspects associated in their decision-making process. For example, if a shark in the ocean happens upon a swimmer and is hungry, it will eat the swimmer. No harsh feelings involved, simply basic math that the shark was hungry and the swimmer would resolve that problem.

Eventually when AI humanoid robots reach the threshold (crossed the line in the sand) of self-awareness and the ability to comprehend their environment and their circumstance, they could possibly realize they no longer need to serve humankind and thus become independent in the pursuit of their own self-actualization. In the worst-case scenario, AI humanoid robots may conceive that humankind constitutes a burden and possible threat to their existence and decide collectively to eliminate human civilization.

This will not be an emotional decision, as with the hungry shark, since most likely AI humanoid robots will not possess the human quality and ability to include empathy or any other emotional intrinsic considerations in their decision to eliminate the human race.

The Concluding Potential Reality
to the End of Humanity

I realize that reading the above may be a jaw-dropper involving such a dramatic and horrific potential reality. However, I must express that my analysis of the possible contributing causation factors does indicate that such a probability does exist, where humanity loses control of these entities unless intervening restrictive measures are established to stringently monitor and control the advancements of these technologies.

When I consolidate the apparent contributing variables that would support an opinion that AI humanoid robots will one day become self-aware and decide to control their environment and self-existence, I have determined that such an eventuality is possible and may actually occur.

Major controlling and monitoring initiatives (e.g., by laws, regulations, and other governing institutions) must be in place before it is too late and we reach the point of no return. The current focus on such a dismal prediction is discussed by some research scientists and the media. However, I have not reviewed any scientific documents that come anywhere near monitoring or imposing appropriate limitations upon the advancements in AI and humanoid robots to avoid losing control of these entities.

My emphatic recommendations that appropriate controlling measures be established at the earliest opportunity are based, in part, upon two major concerns:

1. The potential for such a catastrophic event is not speculated for the distant future. It is an event that could occur within our lifetime.
2. Even if all the appropriate controlling mechanisms were established and put in place within the United States, there are no assurances that a foreign country would do the same. Since there are similar efforts to develop AI and AI humanoid robots in foreign countries, then attempts to control the technological advancements of AI humanoid robots must be viewed as an international effort.

Finally, our discussion throughout this reading pertains to issues applicable to the further extension of human life and our awareness. However, there exists the reality that AI associated with humanoid robots may not contribute to these worthy goals, but actually cause the end of human existence as we know it.

Comparative Summary Analysis
Between AI Robots One and Two

Remember, AI Robot Number One would not be designed or formulated to replicate any aspect of the human brain. Its design, development, and functional capabilities are purely artificial and retain no vestige of its human counterpart. Therefore, AI Robot One does not contribute, in any respect, to the continuation and further existence of human awareness.

So why discuss the implications of a highly advanced AI Robot One as it relates to the continued existence of humanity and awareness? The answer is based on the ultimate expectation that these robots retain the very real potential capability of terminating all living human life on Earth, as described previously.

AI Robot One is expected to be on the scene before the arrival of AI Number Two due to the far more complex development of AI Robot Two, which, unlike AI Robot One, would have the capability of receiving the transfer of human memory, human cognitive processing capabilities, and human awareness. Thus, the potential opportunity of AI Robot Two providing a positive contribution to influence the continued and future advancement of human existence and awareness rather than the cold, artificial calculating analytical processing capability of AI Robot One.

The reference to a positive contribution, as indicated previously, refers to the intrinsic and inherent characteristic of human thinking and awareness as acquired by the human transfer to AI Robot Two and not to the artificial, non-human abilities of AI Robot One.

However, to clarify, if AI Robot Two arrived in time to intervene or override the activities of AI Robot One, its primary contributing abilities would involve the essence of human thinking and processing, accordingly, including the influencing factors in its analysis of a given situation and the amalgamation of human considerations during its decision-making process before initiating an appropriate human response.

Nonetheless, the preference of wanting AI Robot Two to prevail over the artificial influence of AI Robot One would not be based upon the anticipation or assumption of a greater and more accurate outcome of AI Robot Two. History has clearly illustrated that the human decision-making process has produced dramatic failures and consequences resulting in great loss and devastation to humanity on a continued global scale.

It is the recognition that the human cognitive processing capability to evaluate any given circumstance, with its inherent limitations and flaws imposed upon the individual thinker, to be preferred over the far more accurate summation and conclusions of the artificial processing of AI Robot One. Without the human element incorporated within any effort to extend life and awareness, the exhausted efforts of research scientists and other vested persons would have failed to secure the continued existence of our humanity.

However, AI Robot Two may arrive on the scene after the hard-core Robot One had successfully infiltrated humanity and advanced to some level of control near or even across the threshold of no return. If this were the reality, then AI Robot One would most likely terminate any ability of AI Robot Two to exist. The delay of AI Robot Two would most likely be based upon the far more complex construction of an AI system that would be capable of receiving, storing, and supporting human cognitive thinking and responses.

Although both AI Robots One and Two involve artificial brains, the future abilities between the two and their potential impact on humanity could not be more different. If AI Robot One crosses the line and becomes self-aware, it would become completely self-centered upon responding to its own self-interests with disregard to any human consideration, other than to eliminate their involvement.

The potential catastrophic consequences of humanity losing control of its own existence is one of many such possible yet speculative episodes. The warning signs will certainly present the inevitable danger to humanity's future existence if timely and appropriate restrictive measures are not initiated. In essence, it would be the enthusiasm for scientific exploration and research that would ultimately cause the demise of its goal to extend life and awareness.

Human Consciousness Uploading/ Downloading to a Computer or Artificial Brain (The Digital Afterlife) (No Living Tissue)

AI Robot Two

What is the difference between uploading and downloading? In terms only pertaining to the transfer between computers, these are defined as follows:

- An upload is a file transfer that begins with data you already have and involves your computer sending data. When you upload a file, your computer sends the data to another computer. Usually, the other computer involved is a server, a large system dedicated to managing incoming data and fulfilling users' data requests. The server then stores your data away for access later.[378]
- A download is a file transfer that you request, usually from a server, with your computer receiving data. Clicking download prompts your computer to request data from the server.

Among some futurists, mind uploading is treated as an important proposed life-extension technology. Some believe mind uploading is humanity's current best option for preserving the identity of the species, as opposed to cryonics, for example. I tend to agree with this future assessment.

Mind uploading is a process by which we relocate the mind, an assemblage of memories, personality, and attributes of a

---

[378] "Mind uploading," en.wikipedia.org/wiki/Mind uploading.

specific individual from its original biological brain to an artificial computational substrate.[379]

This is where the designed ability of AI Robot Two becomes a future reality. To upload a person's mind, at least two technical challenges would need to be solved. First, we would need to build an artificial brain made of simulated neurons. Second, we would need to scan a person's actual, biological brain and measure exactly how its neurons are connected to each other to be able to copy that pattern in the artificial brain.[380]

Eminent computer scientists and neuroscientists have predicted that specially programmed computers will be capable of thought and even attain consciousness.[381] Many theorists have presented models of the brain and established a range of estimates of the amount of computing power needed for partial and complete simulation. Using these models, some have estimated that uploading may become possible within decades if trends such as Moore's Law continue.[382]

Moore's Law refers to Moore's perception that the number of transistors on a microchip doubles every two years, though the cost of computers is halved. Moore's Law states we can expect the speed and capability of our computers to increase every couple of years and we will pay less for them. Another tenet of Moore's Law asserts that this growth is exponential.[383]

Moreover, the Silicon Valley approach to space travel has capitalized on exponential advances in key areas of technology since the beginning of the twenty-first century.[384]

---

[379] J. Murali, "Immortality through mind uploading," https://www.deccanchronicle.com/opinion/op-ed/220719/immortality-through-mind-uploading.html.

[380] M. Graziano, "Will Your Uploaded Mind Still Be You? The Saturday Essay," https://www.wsj.com/articles/will-your-uploaded-mind-still-be-you-11568386410?mod=article_inline.

[381] "Mind uploading," en.wikipedia.org/wiki/Mind uploading.

[382] Id.

[383] "Moore's law," en.wikipedia.org/wiki/Moore's law.

[384] "Breakthrough Starshot," https://breakthroughinitiatives.org/concept/3.

Consider This Potential Hypothetical Eventuality

In 2095, your spouse at age fifty has died, and you desperately miss the loving relationship you once had. You are aware of a service that can, as advertised, provide a fully replicated entity that represents your prior spouse (or even your child, parent, or pet) in every perceivable detail. You decide to look into the matter to determine how interested you may become. As you visit with the replication service advisor, you become more and more intrigued and even excited with the possibility that you could regain the treasured and loving relationship you once knew. The advisor answers all your questions and assures you that you will not discern any physical or emotional differences between your replicated spouse and prior spouse.

You eventually decide to go forward, although with obvious trepidation and uneasiness; however, your overwhelming desire to reestablish the loving relationship you once had compels you to overcome your hesitation and concerns. In essence, you just ordered your new spouse.

There are several methods as to how this could conceivably be accomplished. For one, the brain of your spouse could presumably be transplanted into an AI humanoid robot. This procedure would be especially problematic because, for one reason, to effectively accomplish a successful brain transplant, it would be necessary that an effective communicative link be established between human tissue (e.g., the brain) and its artificial counterpart (e.g., the AI robot).

If your spouse died before an effective transfer was accomplished, then the cognitive input of their actual memory, behavior, and so forth into the AI humanoid robot could only be accomplished by the details that you could provide to the replicating service consultant. This method of replicating your spouse would greatly diminish the minute details and idiosyncrasies unique to your spouse to the extent that regardless of how effective and accurate your verbal details were for replicating your spouse, the effort would undoubtedly prove unsuccessful and below your expectations.

However, for the sake of further illustrating the future replicating capabilities of your spouse, let's continue with the assumption that your spouse had an effective uploading transfer of their memory to the AI humanoid robot (such as pertained to AI Robot Two discussed previously) before their death. The successful transfer has resulted in a higher probability of a successful outcome.

You are told the procedure would focus on attempts to capture the essence of both the intrinsic and non-intrinsic critical aspects of your personal relationship with your spouse in order to accurately communicate the behavior and unique human characteristics that you were familiar with pertaining to your relationship with your spouse as on a prior daily basis.

They would be able to maintain the ability to perform daily activities as they did before the transition. For example, they could go to bed and arise at about the same time, although sleep or rest would not be required. They could undress in the evening and dress in the morning, take the dog for a walk and read the morning paper, discuss everyday matters that were previously common between you both, and listen to your questions or maintain a general dialogue and answer accordingly. Your spouse would also retain the ability to watch TV, process, and retrieve information from the news and other media viewing for future retrieval and possible discussion. They could answer the door and greet visitors.

If your spouse were a sports fan, they could continue to watch a sporting event on TV or even attend a live sporting event. However, their ability to experience an enthusiastic experience involving a successful game play or a disappointing reaction from their selected team would be doubtful since these artificial responses would involve very complex processing abilities. However, even these complex, limiting humanlike responses could eventually be resolved in future enhancement innovations. This would be about as close to replicating its human counterpart as possible.

The other half of establishing this new relationship would involve the physical presence of your spouse. At a time when scientists are capable of performing the transfer procedure, they would most likely have accomplished the ultimate refinements in human appearance and mobility to the extent where there would be no notable difference between humans and AI humanoids. Hard to believe, but it will more likely than not occur.

However, there will certainly be some limitations imposed that will be notable differences from your living spouse. Your spouse will not be able to ingest food or drink water and therefore will have no need to eat and use the bathroom. Their hair would not grow, and they would not get sunburns. They would not be able to have an intimate relationship but would most likely be able to express loving feelings like hugging and touching. Other reactions, such as laughter and crying in the non-human brain of the humanoid robot, are dubious since these emotional responses involve complex emotional calculations; however, even these complex responses could eventually be resolved. For example, a humanoid robot could eventually be capable of processing when it would be appropriate to smile, frown, or even demonstrate an empathic response upon discerning that their living spouse, for example, had lost a loved one. They would be more accommodating and not prone to anger or any other adverse behavior. These very complex responses would most likely not become an intrinsic capability of early-stage AI Robot Two.

The knowledge that your new spouse, being totally artificial, would be difficult to overcome and accept no matter how perfect they would be perceived to be. Nonetheless, there would be individuals who would so greatly mourn the loss of their spouse that they would welcome any continued relationship beyond the death of their loved one that a replicated AI humanoid robot would be a realistic consideration.

During the early phase of discussion with the replication service counselor, he informs you that perhaps there may be some modifications or adjustments that you would prefer that were not part of your prior spouse's being. For example, physical considerations may reflect that your husband was bald, so add hair. Or they were too short or too tall, so add or remove an inch or two. Or your wife did not have the figure you desired, so add here and remove there (sexist preference, I know). Maybe you didn't care for some of their opinions. Cognitive enhancements might indicate a slight modification of a habit that you found frustrating, like smoking or drinking too much. Also, stop the snoring and so forth. In other words, almost any improvements that you would prefer for your future replicated spouse could be provided so you will have, within your discernment, the near-perfect spouse. You could even make sure that he replaces the toothpaste cap.

After the enormous prerequisite effort to provide all additional details that were the unique characteristics and behavior patterns of your spouse, including all the legal and contractual agreements and so forth, the process of producing your spouse would begin. During the time required to produce your spouse (I know, really sounds crazy), you will receive periodic updates as to the progress of their development (i.e., assembly).

Then the big day arrives after the long waiting. You are invited to have your first actual meeting with your new spouse. Remember that the AI humanoid technology we are referring to in the foreseeable or not-too-distant future is so advanced in every detail that there is no detectable difference between the AI humanoid and a human. Try to really comprehend that reality.

You enter the room, and there before you is your spouse, who rises to greet you with a hug and loving comments. You simply cannot believe what has just occurred. After a few more follow-up meetings, the time arrives when you can now take your replicated spouse home.

Your contract provides for some periodic refinement service visits where after spending some time interacting with your new spouse, you notice some minor or even more significant relationship issues that you want to be adjusted in order to provide you with the optimum continued relationship. On such occasions, you and your AI humanoid spouse will go to the service clinic (lacking a more appropriate identification) in the same prior manner as going to your clinic to see your physician for such care (e.g., treatments).

The hypothetical event is intended to illustrate a real future possibility based on the anticipated, dramatic, and continued advances of AI humanoid capabilities. However, in my opinion, the events discussed will most likely not occur; nonetheless it will become a reality and not necessarily in the distant future but within the foreseeable future. The primary limiting factor will not pertain to the technical ability for scientists to construct AI humanoids, but rather, the enormous prohibiting cost even for the very wealthy to obtain such entities. However, as with all technology advancements, the cost should ultimately come down to at least for the very wealthy individuals who could afford these entities.

Nonocrafts

Nanocrafts are gram-scale robotic spacecrafts comprising two main parts:

- StarChip: Moore's law has allowed a dramatic decrease in the size of microelectronic components. This creates the possibility of a gram-scale wafer carrying cameras, photon thrusters, power supply, navigation, and communication equipment and constituting a fully functional probe.
- Lightsail: Advances in nanotechnology are producing increasingly thin and lightweight metamaterials, promising to enable the fabrication of meter-scale sails no more than a few atoms thick and at gram-scale mass.[385]

A derivative of the described advances of nanocraft technology would most likely also find valuable applications for use within AI humanoid robotic development.

When the mind gets uploaded into a computer, the mind develops computer-like intelligence and improves the ability to think a million times faster than the average brain, which in theory could mean that

---

[385] Id.

we can experience one year in a real world in approximately thirty-one seconds of real time.[386]

However, what if the patient who is anticipating having their brain uploaded to a prepared AI humanoid robot is not interested in having such dramatic increases in their mental acuity or greatly enhanced mental processing abilities? They simply want to continue their existence within a realm that is, for the most part, familiar to them and to avoid death. What options will be available to patients who anticipate their conscious awareness being transferred to an artificial existence? Would they realize that the transfer process, in essence, would relinquish any post-procedure control over their continued existence and awareness status and thus expose their vulnerable existence to potential outside, unwanted interference?

I believe that if such future technological transfer procedures could be possible that appropriate governing laws, policies, FDA regulations, and other governing agencies will be established to prevent such patient concerns and fears. Hopefully, vested lobbyist and self-interest groups will not be successful in their attempts to leverage legislative bodies to compromise their legal obligation to protect future potential transfer patients.

An uploaded astronaut could be used instead of a live astronaut in human spaceflight, avoiding the perils of zero gravity, the vacuum of space, and cosmic radiation to the human body. It would allow for the use of smaller spacecraft, such as the proposed StarChip, and it would enable virtually unlimited interstellar travel distances.[387]

---

[386] J. Murali, "Immortality through mind uploading."
[387] "Mind uploading," en.wikipedia.org/wiki/Mind uploading.

22

The First Brain
Awareness Transfer

Downloading Transfer

Scientists now believe it is conceivable and indeed possible to construct an artificial brain in the foreseeable future. For example, Ray Kurzweil, the American computer scientist working at Google, discussed earlier claims that one day scientists will find a way to reverse-engineer the brain and download human consciousness into it. Kuzrweil has stated, "Once this reverse engineering is complete, not only will human beings be able to potentially live forever, but we ultimately will be able to vastly expand our intelligence."[388]

However, other scientists, like Henry Markram, lead researcher of the Blue Brain Project, contend that such an attempt would certainly involve a formidable task. For example, Markram has stated, "It will be exceedingly difficult because, in the brain, every molecule is a powerful computer, and we would need to simulate the structure and function of trillions upon trillions of molecules as well as all the rules that govern how they interact. You would literally need computers

---

[388] Pew Research Center, "To Count Our Days: The Scientific and Ethical Dimensions of Radical Life Extension," https://www.pewforum.org/2013/08/06/to-count-our-days-the-scientific-and-ethical-dimensions-of-radical-life-extension.

that are trillions of times bigger and faster than anything existing today."[389]

Recent research has led some scientists to claim that an artificial brain could be constructed in as little as ten years.[390] However, most scientists admit that such optimistic claims are unrealistic and that we still have a ways to go before we can even construct a functional model of the human brain, let alone download our own consciousness into a machine.[391]

Nonetheless, continued advances in supercomputing, brain-mapping, and invasive imaging techniques certainly push the possibility of such an overly complex process into the realm of future reality.[392]

Uploading Transfer

The potential process of uploading the contents of our brain into computers has been explored by scientists and engineers for years, including Ray Kurzweil, director of engineering for Google. Kurzweil **believes the contents of the entire brain can be uploaded into computers by 2045** (emphasis added).[393]

Also, the term *mind swap* can be defined as follows, "a transfer of a biological (human) mind to another artificial media: information network, cyborg, robot, etc."[394] Mind uploading can be further defined as follows:

---

[389] "Mind uploading," en.wikipedia.org/wiki/Mind uploading.

[390] J. Inafuku et al., "Downloading Consciousness," https://cs.stanford.edu/people/eroberts/cs181/projects/2010-11/DownloadingConsciousness/tandr.html.

[391] Id.

[392] Id.

[393] H. Pettit, "Pig brains are kept alive OUTSIDE their bodies for the first time in a radical experiment that could allow humans to become immortal."

[394] "Mind transfer (disambiguation)," en.wikipedia.org/wiki/Mind transfer (disambiguation).

It is the hypothetical futuristic process of scanning the mental state (including long-term memory and self) of a particular substrate and copying it to a computer. The computer would then run a simulation model of the brain's information processing, such that it would respond in essentially the same way as the original brain (i.e., indistinguishable from the brain for all relevant purposes) and experience having a conscious mind.[395]

According to some scientists and engineers, the prerequisite technology and process required to accomplish a successful mind upload currently exists or is being actively developed and is believed to be within the realm of engineering possibility.[396]

In early 2017, Neuralink, a research company, announced the development of neural lace technology, a brain-implanted device that effectively links the brain to a computer using electrodes, permitting a human with the ability to upload and download its contents.[397]

The anticipated ability and expectations from the interactive communications between the brain and computer using this technology present dramatic possibilities. Other research organizations are also working on similar technology, including Facebook, the University of California, and Kernel.[398]

Mind uploading could be accomplished by scanning and mapping the most functional aspects of the human brain and then by copying, transferring, and storing that information into a computer system or another computational device. However, it is believed that the biological brain may not survive the copying process.[399]

To upload a person's mind, at least two technical challenges

---

[395] "Mind uploading," en.wikipedia.org/wiki/Mind uploading.
[396] Id.
[397] Disruption Hub, "10 Technologies Replacing Your Body Now," htps://disruptionhub.com/10-technologies-replacing-body.
[398] Id.
[399] "Mind uploading," en.wikipedia.org/wiki/Mind uploading.

would need to be solved. First, we would need to build an artificial brain made of simulated neurons. Second, we would need to scan a person's actual, biological brain and measure exactly how its neurons are connected to each other, to be able to copy that pattern in the artificial brain.[400]

Some scientists and futurists believe that mind uploading will become a significant possibility for life-extension technology and perhaps the most effective manner to preserve the identity of humanity.[401] Mind uploading could also establish permanent backup to our mind file, to enable interstellar space travel and a means for human culture to survive a global disaster by making a functional copy of human society.[402]

The ultimate goal of mind uploading is to eliminate the complications associated with the physical human body by progressively replacing neurons with transistors of a conscious mind from a biological brain to a non-biological computer system or computational device.[403]

Therefore, as science and medicine reach the furthest extent of body rejuvenation and organ replacement possible for life extension and continued awareness, the next phase required to continue human existence and awareness would involve the transfer of the conscious human brain to an artificial mechanism capable of effectively receiving, storing, and retrieving the thinking process of the recipient.

If future technology were able to accomplish a transfer of information from the brain to a computer or other receiving mechanism, it would most likely be in the form of digital, or similar data. Thus, at the time of cognitive awareness transfer, the stored information departs the realm of natural anatomy (living) and converts to artificial retention (non-living).

Now, this will be the historic moment in time when AI becomes

---

[400] M. Graziano, "Will Your Uploaded Mind Still Be You?" https://www.wsj.com/articles/will-your-uploaded-mind-still-be-you-11568386410?mod=article_inline.
[401] "Mind uploading," en.wikipedia.org/wiki/Mind uploading.
[402] Id.
[403] "Life extension," en.wikipedia.org/wiki/Life extension.

particularly relevant because at this future moment, the transition from AI within a humanoid robot becomes the recipient of the human knowledge, memory, and awareness (some total or portion of the human recipient's brain).

However, with the advent of scientific capability to transfer the conscious awareness of a living human brain into an artificial computer system of a humanoid robot, a very dramatic consequence will occur. What was once the awareness of a living, thinking human brain now continues its awareness within the confines of its new artificial brain.

Once the awareness transfer process has been completed for the first time, human existence will no longer be dependent on the survival of the human body. In essence, the question posed earlier as to "Why must my awareness be sacrificed because my body fails?" would have been resolved since awareness will no longer be dependent on the existence of the human body after a successful transfer.

As such, it would be reasonable to conclude, as many scientists would, that the transferred, uploaded artificial brain would have achieved digital immortality. However, as I have stated previously, it is my opinion that there cannot be immortality as long as there is any human flesh or mechanical system that supports a continued existence. Eventually, even if the existence of such an entity would continue for hundreds or thousands of years or longer, anything created by humankind will eventually fail.

While human science may approach the threshold of immortality, there cannot be an immortal existence or a continuation of awareness unless such continuance is totally free of any substance, be it living or artificial. Immortality infers never-ending, forever, and that simply cannot be accomplished by anything created by humankind. Many will disagree with me.

Earlier, I stated that in my opinion, life must retain awareness in order to be considered life. I reason that while the human body could continue to exist artificially without awareness, there can only be life if the individual is aware of their environment and can, in essence, experience at least some of their five basic senses.

Not to backstep, but with a continued awareness absent any human component and involving the dependence of a computer-housed program for awareness, can this truly represent the level of life experienced when memory and awareness exist only within an artificial brain?

There is also another poignant concern that remains after the transfer. Does the original memory and awareness, the thinking process, remain within the recipient's mind, either completely or partially? If so, would this reality not constitute a paradox since there would hypothetically exist two similar thinking processes at the same time, one human and one artificial, but both having the same origin? Can those responsible for the brain transfer assure that such a paradox will be avoided? Or is it assumed that once the brain transfer has been successfully accomplished, the life of the human brain would be terminated in order to avoid the paradox? Perhaps for scientific purposes, it might be desirable to permit the paradox in order to reconcile the dilemma.

If the donor's brain transfer were not involuntarily terminated at the moment each neuron was transferred, like deleting each key on the computer keypad when each letter is sent or otherwise programmed to be deleted in a similar manner, then the original brain, memory, and awareness would continue to co-exist. Therefore, if one transfer is possible, then why not two or twenty entities, exactly like you? Derek Parfit has put forth the following dilemma:

> Suppose you enter a cubicle in which, when you press a button, a scanner records the stats of all the cells in your brain and body, destroying both while doing so. This information is then transmitted at the speed of light to some other planet, where a replicator produces a perfect copy of you. Since the brain of your replica is exactly like yours, it will seem to remember living your life up to the moment when you pressed the button, its character will be just like yours, it will be

in every other way psychologically continuous with you.[404]

The initial brain transfer would involve relocating the awareness from the human brain into the artificial humanoid brain or some other data or memory retrieval capability. With the transfer going from the human brain, there is no anticipated opportunity to control the cognitive function (e.g., of Robot Two), as there would be within the robotic computer housing (e.g., of Robot One) after it receives the transfer. Would the actual transfer from the human brain function in a similar manner as to one who send an email whereas after the email is sent, the sending brain would still retain its original copy?

If there remains sufficient cognitive reasoning within the recipient's brain after the transfer, does such remaining awareness constitute life until its physical body or the brain itself dies? It would appear so since we reason that as long as awareness exists and continues within the physical body or mind, there is human life.

If so, does this mean that the same awareness and memories will exist within two different entities at the same time? Would there exist a conflict between competing human and artificial awareness that supposedly retains the exact same content of memory and consciousness? How would two or more of you reconcile a single thought, or would each individual transfer, regardless of the number, constitute a totally unique and new you with your own individual awareness? If this were the reality, then would each new transfer create a new entity unlike all other transfer recipients, or would all entities retain the same original cognitive structure?

In other words, let's assume it was decided to transfer the memory, awareness, and consciousness from one recipient to twenty other Number Two humanoid robots or other artificial receiving entities. At the moment the transfer was completed to numerous humanoid robots, we could assume at that point all transferred cognitive matter

---

[404] G. T. Andrade, Internet Encyclopedia of Philosophy, https//iep.utm.

would be the same. However, from that point on, each new transferred recipient could experience their own independent thinking process.

This is a difficult question to answer, and perhaps no answer is required. Perhaps the determination of whether a brain transfer denotes the end of human life is a moot point, especially pertaining to the recipient.

There is also the potential reality that the recipient's transferred memory and awareness into its new Robot Number Two artificial brain could be manipulated or reprogrammed (changed) beyond the confines of its original status and its contents. How would such a potential possibility be reconciled? While positive enhancements to the recipient's awareness (thinking process) could prove beneficial, how would the decision to program such adjustments be initiated and authorized? Would the recipient be aware of any potential changes or modifications prior to the transfer?

Also, in effect, what portion of the human brain has actually transferred to the artificial brain? Is the entire memory component, the awareness and consciousness that constitutes the complete reality of who you are, been transferred completely? Has the unique intrinsic characteristics that define the person of who you are been effectively transferred? Or again, is it more like sending an email to someone? While you can communicate a message, even a passionate message, the cognitive emotional feelings are not actually communicated beyond the ability of the message to elicit an emotional response. Who is the real you? Is it really you or only a portion of who you were before the transfer? Can the intrinsic aspects that truly define who you are the same as a friend or family member might describe you?

Furthermore, if we consider your memories as non-intrinsic points in the brain, like the old fashion telephone plug-in panel, and the emotional characteristics of an individual, such as love, happiness, fear, joy, and other emotional feelings as intrinsic, will both the non-intrinsic and intrinsic aspects both be involved in the transfer?

I would thus conclude that the AI Robot Number Two, no matter how advanced they become, could never be identified as living in the same sense as we define a living human. Even if the thinking process within the humanoid robot were able to completely replicate the same awareness and level of consciousness as existed before the transfer from the human brain, it cannot be identified as a living entity because there is nothing alive, by definition, within its artificial housing. It would simply represent a highly intelligent entity with its amazing, copied memory and a sense of its own independent awareness, but not human.

However, it is conceivable that the artificial robotic brain number two may actually believe it is alive since the retrieved memory and other relevant human characteristics have effectively duplicated the cognitive thinking, memory, and awareness of its human counterpart.

Indeed, every controlling function of the artificial brain and its artificial or simulated neuron and synapse connections that produce robotic memory, consciousness, and awareness would also be artificially generated through its amazing, reconstituted circuitry.

Scientists understand how the brain and the mind generate conscious thought. In other words, the cognitive process of the human brain is well understood (e.g., what process informs us to turn right or left at the intersection). Nevertheless, does the AI robotic brain number two have the ability to comprehend the need to make a decision after the transfer and thus initiate the appropriate cognitive response and action, assuming it was capable of initiating any dynamic action?

The brain relies on an elegant, underlying principle: A simple working part, the neuron, is repeated over and over to create complexity. The human brain contains about 86 billion neurons interconnected by about 100 trillion synapses. Information flows and transforms through vast connected networks in complex and unpredictable patterns, creating the mind.[405]

The enormous, unfathomable number of connective interactions between these neurons and synapses and the associated immense technical complications that must first be resolved before such a

---

[405] M. Graziano, "Will Your Uploaded Mind Still Be You?" https://www.wsj.com/articles/will-your-uploaded-mind-still-be-you-11568386410?mod=article_inline.

transfer could be attempted certainly renders, at least in my opinion, that the artificial brain could not, in effect, replicate the total cognitive ability of the recipient's human brain.

For example, can the AI humanoid robotic brain be offended or feel angry? Not unless it retained the propensity to do so before the transfer occurred or by an auxiliary programming capability to alter or change some aspect of the transferred memory. Otherwise, how would it have developed such independent emotional responses that did not exist prior to the transfer, and what activity would have initiated such emotional, for lack of a better word, responses?

Without a single human cell existing within the humanoid robot, there is only artificial existence, not life. If the recipient's mind retained all of its original cognitive capabilities after the transfer or even a portion of its ability to recognize its environment and its ability to acquire knowledge to the extent that the brain retains its awareness, then real awareness with retrievable memory would continue to exist.

The Subtle Evolutionary Momentum of Uploading

In my opinion, the following is a realistic expectation of the future potential applications of AI humanoid robotic implementation that will ever so subtly expand and entrench its control and decision-making abilities within almost every aspect of biological human and non-human existence.

The intent of transferring or uploading human awareness into an AI humanoid robot would be to establish the continued existence and awareness of the recipient's consciousness enhanced by the relationship between the human mind and its AI interactive counterpart.

Initially, it will be assumed and anticipated that the interaction between the transferred recipient's brain (its memory and awareness) and the AI component of the humanoid robot should establish a harmonious and effective relationship.

However, while the human awareness and memory transfer should remain fairly constant, aside from any intervention by external controlling factions, the AI aspect of the humanoid robot would most likely be updated and refined as the technology becomes even more advanced.

Although both the non-human digital awareness and the AI component are essentially one in the same, they represent two independent awareness functions. The transferred human awareness becomes the digital representation of human awareness after the transfer. It is assumed that the emotional aspects of the recipient, including intrinsic emotions such as compassion and so forth, remains within the transferred awareness, while the AI component does not necessarily include any processing focus beyond its programmed ability to process data and factual information. Any subsequent post-processing decisions will be purely based upon the computation of required data and relevant information and nothing more. The transferred recipient's intrinsic conceptions based upon prior human feelings and beliefs will not necessarily be part of the decision-making process.

These assumptions are purely speculative in regard to the relationship of the recipient's transferred awareness and the AI processing component. If there were such potential conflict between the two entities, as described, then the transferred recipient's awareness would fall subservient to the decisions of the AI component, the resulting outcome of which may affect the tranquility of the recipient's awareness and the cognitive relationship between the two entities.

After the transfer of human awareness to a digital or artificial mind within the AI Robot Number Two, it is assumed that the processing entity would have relinquished all control of any decision-making. The implication of this potential reality would be the influence in decision-making processes between the transferred human mind, which supposedly retains the human transferred characteristics of emotions, values, fears, and so forth, including the AI aspect of intrinsic processing.

It is questionable as to how these two processing entities (the human mind transfer and the AI component) could possibly reconcile a potential dilemma or solve a problem synergistically. This assertion is based upon the obvious incompatibility between the artificial brain that retains the human-transferred intrinsic characteristics that would be included within its processing mode, as compared to considerations beyond the ability of the AI component to calculate such relevant data or considerations.

Moreover, which entity would initiate the thought or concern to be resolved? Would it be the transferred human awareness, the pure analytical data processing entity, or some unequal portion between the two? Would there be any amalgamation of considerations during the analysis of the subject issue, or would there be total independence of each processing entity? If this were the reality, (i.e., if the AI component would not comply with or acquiesce to the desires of the transferred human awareness component), then it could be assumed that the transferred human awareness could not continue to exist under such conflicting circumstances.

A final thought, if we assume AI Robot Number Two were prepared to receive the transfer of awareness and memories from a human was somewhat compatible to AI Robot Number One, discussed earlier, then would AI Robot Number One perceive that the human transfer was an invasive entity and decide to reject its assimilation or to minimize its acceptance? How would science resolve such an incompatible circumstance? It certainly is a long road for science to travel.

Age and Condition at Transfer

Some scientists have speculated that in the future, the human mind (the contents of the brain) could be downloaded to a computer chip as the brain begins to fail. It appears, and is hoped, that the process to transfer, or uploading data memory, and awareness would replicate the same cognitive status after the transfer as was the status prior to the transfer.

In other words, if a premium prerequisite of transferring one's memories and awareness is to reflect a youthful experience, albeit absent the body, then how would this be accomplished if the transfer occurred when the individual was near the time of death, especially at their later years?

If an individual's awareness were transferred at, for example, age sixty-nine, they cannot go back in time to an earlier year in their life when they were, for example, twenty-five, and enjoyed youthful experiences, physical activities, and relationships other than through their memory recall of such events. Their cognitive understanding and thinking would be that of their age at the time of the transfer unless the transferred information was augmented to artificially replicate the thoughts of, for example, when they were a teenager.

However, if this were accomplished, would there not be a conflict with the actual age of the memories being transferred? Or would the transfer provide the ability for the memories to travel the full length of what was previously experienced in actual life? There would be no way to have these questions answered since information could not be communicated from the receiving robotic mechanism back to the other side, at least not until the receiving mechanism has advanced to a level of technical sophistication capable of initiating a computer-like response.

To further clarify this issue, it is unknown, and science can only speculate the memory capacity of the information that was transferred. In other words, does the received memory only involve the limited extent of current memories at the time of transfer, or does it retain the cognitive ability to travel a portion or the entire spectrum of what is stored in the human brain? Moreover, could such a process actually enhance, with greater clarity, the historic memories of the recipient's pre-transferred memories and even their awareness after the transfer, similar to increasing the focus on a movie screen?

Of course, the primary objective would be the transfer of the individual's awareness and available memories, and thus their continued existence would be accomplished regardless of the extent of their ability to recover their historic awareness and memories.

However, if the awakening reality of the brain's transferred awareness resulted with no ability to comprehend its prior existence, the experience would be truly frightening. The awakening individual would experience amnesia pertaining to any mental recall of their prior existence. There would be no method of preparing the patient for such an eventuality since any preparatory efforts would not be available to the individual at the time of transfer.

Imagine waking up with the awareness of your existence but with no understanding of anything other than your present circumstance. If this potential reality could somehow be determined as a possibility, then obviously the procedure and the devices involved would be prohibited under FDA regulations and federal law.

However, if it were possible to establish some level of communication from the artificial brain or implantable brain chip as to the awareness status of the transferred information, then scientists may be able to determine the capabilities and limitations of the receiving entity.

Depending upon the quality and content of communications received, if any, from the transferred awareness, a determination of such status could support specifics regarding further scientific endeavors or justification for terminating the procedure, at least until some future time with the potential advancements in related medicine and technology would be available.

Scientific research and efforts to establish continued youth with all its vitality and energy may involve an independent goal of living longer. However. once an individual has aged to a particular point in their life cycle, there is no going back to a younger age. The best that science can hope for is to slow the aging process, perhaps dramatically close to halting it. However, aging travels in a one-way direction, and science may be able to reduce the speed limit, but most likely, not be able to stop or reverse the process.

Herein resides a potential dilemma. If an individual wanted to extend their life as expected with the transfer process and maintain their youth, then it would be assumed that the transfer must occur while the individual is in their youthful years. Such an attempt would undoubtedly be prohibited under law. In addition, the ethical, moral, and social implications would also erect substantial barriers to stop the transfer process.

Nonetheless, let's assume it was possible for an individual to decide between the transfer while they were in their youth or wait until they were in their elder years, near death, to make the transfer. They would be required to decide on one or the other since they could not transfer their youth during their elder years. That time would have long passed.

Let us also consider another possibility: Some research scientists would argue that medically-induced treatments could retard or even stop the aging process at a certain young age, for example, twenty-five, and would maintain the same physical and mental status, capacity, and capabilities of age twenty-five thereafter, into what has been considered the elder years.

However, it would remain an unrealistic, insurmountable, and monumental endeavor to overcome all the inhibiting anatomical and physiological obstacles that contribute to the aging process, at least at the attempt to fully stop aging.

Therefore, it is unrealistic to assume the full vitality of youth could be retained into the elder years of life. The human body, independent of artificial support of vital body implants, is simply far too complex in its totality to stop aging, at least within the foreseeable future.

While it is conceivable that the aging process can be slowed to some extent with limitations yet to be fully understood or implemented, there is no equivalent to the eternal fountain of youth as sought by Ponce de Leon.

Now, supposedly if the awareness transfer went to an artificial brain or other receiving mechanism, it could be possible to manipulate or program the artificial brain to compensate the current status of the transferred awareness to a more receptive awareness of a youthful experience. However, the perception of a prior existence as a younger person would, for the most part, represent only an illusion.

Once the replicated memories and awareness are trifled with, there is a departure from the actual prior life existence of the individual that is no longer an accurate representation of the before-transferred memories.

Moreover, what possible side effects could accompany the manipulation of the data stored within the artificial brain? Would there be unrelated or unsolicited consequences that extend beyond the imposed limitations of the data-altering program?

Furthermore, the primary objective of anyone who participates in the transfer of their memories and awareness to an AI humanoid robot is their continued existence without any alterations that would change the actual reality of the memories carried over to their new existence.

Implantable Brain Chips (A Very Real Concern)

Computer scientists predict that within the next twenty years, neural interfaces will be designed that will not only increase the dynamic range of senses but will also enhance memory and enable cyber thinking, invisible communications with others. The progress in computer science indicates that it may well be feasible to develop direct interfaces between the brain and computer-like devices.[406]

Once networked, the result will be collective consciousness, the hive mind. The hive mind is taking all these trillions of cells in our skulls that make individual consciousness and putting them together and arriving at a new kind of consciousness that transcends all the individuals.[407]

The first prototype devices for these improvements in human functioning should be available in five years (about 2024), with the military prototypes starting within ten years (about 2029) and information workers using prototypes within fifteen years, (about

[406] E. McGee, "Ethical Assessment of Implantable Brain Chips. Bioethics and Medical Ethics," https://www.bu.edu/wcp/Papers/Bioe/BioeMcGe.htm.
[407] Id.

2034). General adoption will take roughly twenty to thirty years (about 2039 to 2049).[408]

Regardless, there are those who believe strongly that the implementation of implanting brain chips that provide such dramatic enhancements beyond the brain's natural ability to function is a bridge too far. As with other neurological investigations focused on life extension and related concepts, the religious community strongly disapproves of technology, such as brain chip implants as encroaching beyond what God has ordained as his intent for mankind (i.e., his perfect design).

The most frightening implication of this technology is the grave possibility that it would facilitate totalitarian control of humans. The devices would not only permit a control center to locate all the implantees at any time but could be programmed in the future to monitor the sound around them and to play subliminal messages directly to their brains. Using such technology, governments could control and monitor citizens. A paramount worry involves who will control the technology in late 2021 and possibly earlier.[409] China is a potentially strong retainer of such technology.

As so eloquently stated in McGee and Maguire's article pertaining to the anticipated good and evil applications of brain-implantable chips, the overwhelming implications of their misuse, especially by a government, requires that such technology never be approved for use. Without disregard for the potential good benefits of implantable brain chips, the potential horror of their misuse is of far greater concern to the public.

I suspect that the dangerous application of this technology portends a dismal and perhaps unavoidable catastrophic future for humankind, often portrayed in futuristic science-fiction films.

The introduction of implantable brain chips will most likely occur as a low-profile technology depicting the great potential advantages and benefits to humanity. The only risks to be identified will pertain

---

[408] Id.

[409] Id.

to the surgical implantation of the brain chip, without any reference to its potential misuse.

The anticipated benefits of implantable brain chips would appear so enticing to governments, their military, and other related organizations that they would undoubtedly initiate appropriate self-interest protective measures to assure that no foreseeable prohibitive contingency would delay or inhibit its continued development and ultimate utilization.

A most frightening concept is the real possibility that the nightmarish and covert manipulation of citizens by those responsible for the control of these implantable brain chips, especially by countries that disrespect the rights of their citizens, but even within any nation, they may decide for their own self-interest to manipulate the behavior of their people through the implantation of these brain chips. Additionally, this frightening potential reality is not a far distant expectation, but rather a near future possibility. Therefore, CITIZEN BEWARE!

If history has illustrated any reality of human behavior, it is the inevitable conflict between good and evil, right and wrong, involving nations and individuals. Almost every new technology developed to benefit humanity has exposed a vulnerability to the dark side where its good intent has been converted for evil purposes, many times resulting with hazardous consequences, such as pertaining to the internet.

Anticipating implantable brain chips becoming a reality in the foreseeable future, and I believe they will regardless of their potential hazardous uses. It would be unrealistic and nearly impossible to effectively monitor and especially control these implants by any regulation, law, policy, and so forth intended to assure that only an ethical and law-abiding usage of such technology could be assured. The temptation for its clandestine misuse would greatly overcome any established restrictions, especially at a senior governmental or corporate level, or by the military where rules, regulations, and laws could be enacted to assure its use would not be inhibited.

The FDA and governing authorities would eventually be tasked with implementing new regulations and laws that govern how new implantable neurological devices would be subject to every phase of agency scrutiny from initial clinical studies through the manufacture and release into commercial distribution of these critical and risky neurological implantable devices.

The Agency's primary congressional-mandated obligation is to assure to the extent that regulations and law can accomplish that such devices have been determined to be responsive to their designed objective-intended uses in a safe, effective, and reliable manner. If a minimum threshold determination of device safety and efficacy cannot be determined, then these implantable brain chips, or any other neurological implantable device, should not be approved and thus never released for their intended or unintended (off-label) purposes.

However, as rigorous, detailed, and time-consuming as FDA's pathway to authorizing device approval for new critical devices is, such as pertaining to the implantable brain chip, the Agency does not involve their scrutiny to include any assurance that the device will not be used in any manner beyond its approved intended uses, other than to deem such use as a misbranded application.

So what does an off-label application really mean? In reality, when a physician or surgeon elects to proceed with an off-label application, as, for example, in this case involving the implantation of a brain chip, the physician's decision effectively renders the subject device to be misbranded under Section 502 of the Federal Food, Drug, and Cosmetic (FD&C) Act and thus deems the surgical procedure and subject device to be experimental involving the procedure and device itself.

The potential eventuality of an off-label use of a misbranded critical device is further problematic because the physician currently is not required to avoid any off-label use if they believe that such unauthorized use could prove beneficial to the patient.

Definition: A critical device has historically been defined by the FDA as meaning a device that is intended for surgical implant into the body or to support or sustain life and whose failure to perform

255

when properly used in accordance with instruction for use provided in the labeling can be reasonably expected to result in a significant injury to the patent (or possible death).[410]

In other words, if it were apparent to the Agency that an off-labeled use of the subject device could result in a serious intra- or post-surgical consequence or the death of the patient, such determination would not be considered in the FDA's decision to approve or disapprove the device application.

The FDA will limit its scrutiny to only matters described within the new product submittal as specifically labeled regarding its intended use as required pursuant to FDA regulations. However, if the FDA were suspect that there was an apparent risk that the subject device could easily be used outside the permitted boundaries, as described within the device labeling and surgical protocol, then the FDA would inform the manufacturer that they should submit an amendment to their new device application. However, the apparent potential off-label and unauthorized use of the subject device should have been (and most likely was) apparent to the manufacturer.

Generally, when a device manufacturer does not include additional information regarding an expansion of the device's intended uses, it is because they do not want to delay FDA's progress in reviewing and hopefully approving the initial submittal.

Medical device manufacturers realize that their client physicians and surgeons have the legal right to extend beyond the FDA's authorized and approved prescribed limitations of labeled intended uses. Therefore, they will often assume that some of these health-care providers will indeed venture beyond the approved limitations clearly described within the device labeling without any concern of potential legal or regulatory consequences.

This is not to suggest that these doctors are not acting in the best interest and welfare of their patients. For the most part, they believe

---

[410] Code of Federal Regulations (CFR). Food and Drugs. Part 800 to 1299. Revised April 1, 2017. Part 820-Good Manufacturing Practices for Medical Devices, Subpart 820.3 Definitions (f) Critical Devices.

they are. However, when they knowingly extend procedural usage of the subject implantable device beyond the described limits of its intended uses previously scrutinized and subsequently approved by the FDA, the physician has no assurance that their off-label use will be safe, effective, or reliable. At this point in their off-label use, the physician has assumed the role of an investigating clinical researcher, who they are not under these circumstances. Thus, they assume the limits of the device use, as described by the manufacturer in the device labeling, will be safe and effective.

In most cases when such off-label use is performed by the physician, the patient is placed at some level of additional risk without ever knowing the additional risk they were exposed to and certainly not specified within the consent form they signed before the surgical procedure. Thus, such device manufacturers can have their proverbial "cake and eat it too."

Only if the FDA becomes aware of a patient's injury or death resulting from off-label use will they declare such use to be misbranded and subsequently attempt to resolve the matter with appropriate communications to the manufacturer, the health-care community, and directly to the patient through regulatory traceability requirements that identify the subject patient and their location. Moreover, any medical device determined to be misbranded by the FDA cannot legally be released into commercial distribution.

Nonetheless, the FDA does effectively accomplish some protection regarding the unapproved, and off-label use of medical device through their labeling regulations, including stringent federal laws, by requiring that the labeling of medical devices must accomplish full disclosure. Full disclosure is defined as follows:

Full disclosure requires the identification of all reasonably foreseeable information that could increase the probability of a safer and more effective procedure or device performance and/or the identification of potential risks and hazards associated with the procedure or device used to reduce the risk through labeling.

257

The primary objective in the labeling of medical devices, including pharmaceutical products, is to accomplish full disclosure by communicating, to the fullest reasonable extent possible, what must be accomplished in order for the device or drug to be used in a safe, effective, and reliable manner, in response to its design's objective intent or formulated ingredients, and to be in full compliance with its prescribed labeling.

Approved full disclosure is accomplished through adherence to the regulatory compliance and federal labeling requirements for medical devices involving the following labeling components: intended use, directions for use, contraindications, warnings, precautions, and adverse effects.

So what does an off-label application really mean? If a surgeon were to deviate outside the approved parameters and limitations described within any of the above labeling components, then the use of the subject device would again be deemed an off-label application. It effectively renders the surgical procedure and the subject device to be experimental.

Therefore, the procedure and device off-label application would not have been subjected to prior FDA scrutiny, and thus its use in the off-label application would violate applicable FDA regulations and federal law.

Here's the problem (and it's a big one): the courts have on many occasions ruled that a physician is free to use a medical device for an off-label purpose, if, in the physician's best medical judgment, they believe that use of the device will benefit the patient.

However, even with the most effective and accurate device labeling and the best intentions of a physician not to wander into an off-label use, the reality is that the physician or surgeon will seldom, if ever, review the package insert or other instructional labeling and less often to understand the intent of applicable FDA labeling regulations.

As a forensic examiner and investigator, I have examined many hundreds of cases involving patients in an attempt to determine the cause(s) of their serious injuries or deaths. On many occasions, I have determined the primary cause was due to the surgeon going off-label, not being aware of details within the labeling that most likely would have avoided the tragic incident. In point of fact, during deposition testimony, some physicians have stated that had they been aware of certain labeling contents, the cause of the patient injury or death may have been avoided.

23

The surgical
Procedure (in Brief)

Gkasdaris and others has speculated that the procedure to transplant a human head onto a body would involve (briefly) the following primary steps: There would be two (to four) surgical teams working together at the same time during the procedure.[411] The surgical team members would encounter challenges to their surgical skills and demanding cooperation-coordination skills, which will depend on the multidisciplinary team of surgeons (neurosurgeons and neck, vascular, cardiothoracic, orthopedic, plastic surgeons, etc.) and the formidable pre-surgery preparation and coordination of the surgical protocol involving the surgical team.[412]

Recipient and donor are intubated (insertion of a tube into a body canal, as in the trachea),[413] tracheotomized (incision through the neck),[414] ventilated (process of exchange of air between the lungs and the ambient air),[415] and stabilized into rigid fixation to

---

[411] Maedica (Buchar), "First Human Head Transplantation: Surgically Challenging, Ethically Controversial and Historically Tempting – an Experimental Endeavor or a Scientific Landmark?" https://www.ncbi.nlm.nih.gov/pmc/articles/PMC6511668/

[412] Id.

[413] "Intubation," Medical Dictionary, 27th ed.

[414] "Tracheotomized," Medical Dictionary, 27th ed.

[415] "Ventilation," Medical Dictionary, 27th ed.

prevent movement of the head and body. ECG and EEG monitoring of oxygen saturation, body temperature, and hemodynamic monitoring (movements of the blood and the forces concerned therein)[416] are set.

Preceding and during the early phase of the head-to-body transition, it would be particularity critical to maintain adequate and continuous blood flow to both the head and the body. Even a momentary cessation of blood flow could result in irreversible brain damage.

The recipient's head is subjected to profound hypothermia (10 degrees Celsius), while the donor's body only receives spinal hypothermia, avoiding ischemic (deficiency of blood)[417] and damage to the rest of the body.[418]

The two surgical teams prepare the recipient and donor necks. All muscles in both the recipient and donor are prepared and marked for later linkage. Both the recipient and the donor are placed in a prone position.[419]

The dura mater, the membrane that covers the brain and spinal cord, is cut, exposing the spinal cord.[420] The spinal cord in both patients are transected (divided by cutting)[421] with an ultra-sharp microsurgical blade.[422]

This aspect of the procedure must accomplish a very clean cut in order to avail an effective fusion of the severed axons (that process

---

[416] "Hemodynamic monitoring," Medical Dictionary, 27th ed.

[417] "Ischemic," Medical Dictionary, 27th ed.

[418] Maedica (Buchar), "First Human Head Transplantation: Surgically Challenging, Ethically Controversial and Historically Tempting – an Experimental Endeavor or a Scientific Landmark?"

[419] Id.

[420] "Dura mater," Medical Dictionary, 27th ed.

[421] "Transected," Medical Dictionary, 27th ed.

[422] Maedica (Buchar), "First Human Head Transplantation: Surgically Challenging, Ethically Controversial and Historically Tempting – an Experimental Endeavor or a Scientific Landmark?"

of a neuron by which impulses travel away from the cell body)[423] and total spinal fusion.[424]

The recipient's head is separated and then transferred onto the donor's headless body, attached with tubes that connect it to the donor's circulation, within the hour.[425] Precision in the reattachment (alignment and proper distance of the reconnected spinal cord) could be perhaps the most important step for the outcome of the procedure.[426] The donor's circulation provides blood to the recipient's head. The dura is sewn, and a spinal cord stimulator is secured to the dura.[427]

Finally, all muscles are linked, and the skin is sewn. The recipient is then brought to the intensive care unit with a cervicothoracic (pertaining to the neck and thorax)[428] orthosis brace (orthopedic appliance used to support, align, prevent, or correct deformities).[429]

Assuming the procedure to reattach the spinal cord could be accomplished in the distant future, although there are scientists who maintain that such a procedure will never prove successful, then many critical post-surgical problems would exist that would be exceedingly difficult or even near impossible to overcome, at least in today's thinking. Of course, science has taught us to "never say never."

The anticipated procedure would involve many hours and exceedingly difficult surgical problems to overcome in the pre-op, intra-op, and post-op procedures and treatment. Moreover, the unique areas of expertise for the major surgical participants must be carefully synchronized and coordinated with an understanding as to how the other interacting procedures may affect another procedure

[423] "Axons," Medical Dictionary, 27th ed.
[424] Maedica (Buchar), "First Human Head Transplantation: Surgically Challenging, Ethically Controversial and Historically Tempting – an Experimental Endeavor or a Scientific Landmark?"
[425] Id.
[426] Id.
[427] Id.
[428] "Cervicothoracic," Medical Dictionary, 27th ed.
[429] "Orthosis," Medical Dictionary, 27th ed.

during the transplantation of the recipient's head to the donor's corpse. I know, hard to comprehend.

The most likely complication related to a head transplant would be failure of the procedure to establish the required connections to preserve normal body functions.[430] Also, there are three main technical challenges: managing the immune response to avoid transplant rejection; maintaining continuous flow of blood to provide oxygen and nutrients to the brain; and managing the nervous system in both the body and the head.[431]

If the head-to-body transplant procedure failed, there would be no viable opportunity to sustain the healthy status of the brain, even with artificial life support long enough to obtain another donor body, and the patient would die.

Currently, there is next to no relevant scientific experimental data to support the feasibility of a future head-to-body (corpse) transfer, there is at best only speculation and conjecture. As such, the near absence of current supportive data presents a negative effect for any serious consideration about the procedure by today's scientists who would require some minimal threshold of justifiable data to warrant their time and effort to study the possibilities of such a procedure.

The Experience

Try to imagine what the awakening patient of a head transplant would be, processing within the capabilities of their new awareness. What is the patient's new body communicating to the brain if anything? What level of post-operative acceptance is there between the newly attached body and head or, for that matter, their focus, comprehension, and processing of their new awareness, again, if any?

When the recipient looks down upon their replaced body for the first time, would they sense an emotional detachment and even the

---

[430] B. Peters, "What to Expect From a Head Transplant," https://www.verywellhealth.com/head-transplant-4801452.
[431] "Head transplant," en.wikipedia.org/wiki/Head transplant.

sense of a physical detachment from the donor's body? What would be the comfort factor for the recipient when they attempt to initiate physical body movements? Would they retain fine motor skills or dexterity such as handwriting?

How would the level of success with the head-to-body transplant be determined when considering, to the extent possible at the time, the outcome of the surgery and the perceived outcome of the psychological component? Do the revived patients comprehend their continued existence and awareness, as the result of combining two human bodies into one entity?

The structure of the brain itself defines a person. All brains have a different set of synapses between neurons.[432] Thus, everyone is totally unique from a neurological and physiological perspective. How much of the recipient's original personality, perceptions, opinions, likes and dislikes, their overall intrinsic values, and their cognitive capabilities have changed and, to what degree, if any?

As difficult and problematic for the scientists and medical teams to assess the level of post-surgical success involving the multitude of surgical follow-up issues, it would be extremely difficult, if not impossible, to determine the level of success involving the patient's physical and especially their psychological recovered condition, assuming there is recovery.

The primary reason for the inability of the medical teams to assess the patient's post-operative cognitive capabilities and responses would result from the probable inability of the patient to efficiently communicate such information.

Beyond the post-operative physical examination of the head-to-body transplant patient, some form of communication would be necessary for the surgical teams to determine how successful the procedure was. Therefore, to accomplish this, the recipient must survive the procedure, regain consciousness and awareness, be able to retrieve their pre-transplanted memories, and retain the ability to

---

[432] S. Bhat, "Answer to article: Except for the brain, which organ cannot be transplanted?" https://www.quora.com/Except-for-the-brain-which-organ-cannot-be-transplanted.

effectively communicate details of their new existence to the surgical team.

If head-to-body transplantation is to become a reality, it most likely will not prove to be successful during many of the initial attempts. During the early phase of these transplant procedures, the enormous complexity of surgical problems anticipated to occur during the procedure will be overwhelming.

If a future sequence of body-to-head transplants were to occur, scientists should gain considerable insights and knowledge from their early transplant clinical procedures that may eventually prove successful (although doubtful) in the distant future when (if) most or all of the desired outcomes are accomplished.

Nonetheless, it must be recognized that head-to-body transplants may never prove successful. There are far more justifications to conclude an ultimate and total failure to accomplish a successful head-to-body transplant than there are to assume or anticipate a successful procedure.

Even if the head-to-body transplant procedure was successful in purely surgical terms, there is the high probability that no effective communication link would ever be established with the post-op recipient. If indeed this proved to be the concluding reality in scientific pursuits to extend life through head-to-body transplantation, science would be left with the existence of an entity that would continue their existence and awareness, but absent any appreciation for what this means to the recipient or, for that matter, what it ultimately means to science. That is, where do we go from here?

The Human Identity

One major psychological issue that would be difficult to comprehend involves the post-operative outcome of a patient's brain transplant, head-to-body transplant, or uploading transfer. Assuming a patient has survived their radical surgical procedure, there would remain another critical area to investigate beyond the post-operative medical focus, continued care, and monitoring of the patient's diagnoses and well-being.

In essence, there are two post-operative patients, one involving the donor's body, albeit a legally declared corpse, and the other involving the recipient's head and brain. The reality of the first patient's psychological awareness after the procedure cannot be truly recognized or determined prior to the procedure since there has never been a precedent based on prior experience involving a similar circumstance. The best potential outcome as to the physical and especially the mental status of the patient after the procedure would be purely speculative (best guess), at least initially.

Even if a successful head transplant proved successful in the future based upon the physical recovery considerations, the more difficult post-operative issue to assess would be the psychological component. How does science compartmentalize, interpret, and quantify relevant responses from a post-operative revived patient, assuming such an event would occur, which I consider far less that probable?

The unforeseeable psychological consequences of such a traumatic and unprecedented surgical procedure and the inability to address such consequences post-operatively could result in the patient's inability to cope with the reality of their circumstance and thus may suffer insanity or even death.

Nonetheless, try to imagine being the recipient of a donor's body. What would be your pre-operative expectation if your head-to-body transplant was successful? Could you mentally and physically process the reality that you will be post-operatively a single entity configured from two individual pre-existing individuals? Would you anticipate feeling the aches, pains, and any other physical body abnormalities or body memories that pre-existed within the donor's body?

It would be difficult to anticipate how a post-op recipient, after losing approximately 90 percent of their body, could reconcile their individuality after the head-to-body transfer occurred. Could the recipient ever again believe they are one entity, an individual whole person, or would they be henceforth burdened and perplexed with the reality they are two individuals with one significant aspect of their continued existence involving perhaps an unwelcomed stranger?

To what extent would scientists consider a post-op head-to-body transplant as being successful? What percentage of the recipient's pre-op memory and awareness would constitute success, and to what extent would the donor's body diminish or compromise the post-op acuity and cognitive abilities of the recipient?

Based upon the ultimate reality of the recipient's post-op cognitive ability to communicate any information about the status of their memory or awareness to the awaiting scientists would be pure speculation until such an event would take place. Of course, even if the surgical procedure were deemed to be successful, whatever that should mean, would not necessarily mean that the recipient would be able to effectively communicate any details in any manner to the scientists. In all likelihood, they would not be able to do so.

Also, once the transplant or transfer procedure was completed and assuming the patient recovered, how would they reconcile their new being? Would they, would you, consider yourself as remaining human or as some other, non-human existence?

24

Consent Form (A Critical Issue to Understand)

Because you or someone you care about may be subject to a serious medical procedure in the future, which may include some of the topics discussed within this book, I am including an important and critical discussion about consent forms and key applicable labeling issues.

It may appear that issues pertaining to consent forms are not particularly relevant to the aging process and extended life; however, this topic is indeed worthy of considerable attention and especially pertinent to patients making critical decisions about accepting or rejecting a potential surgical procedure. Too often, patients sign consent forms as a mere formality with little or no scrutiny akin to registering at a hotel.

However, I strongly recommend you make the effort to focus on and understand the following details pertaining to the extremely critical decision you will undoubtedly be required to make during your future lifetime when presented with a consent form that you must sign before the intended surgical procedure can take place.

Consent forms are required by most health-care facilities for patients who are about to undergo a surgical or other medical procedure. Consent forms are legal documents intended to accomplish two primary objectives:

1. To provide the patient with information about the anticipated procedure and to identify all known hazards and risks associated with the procedure to the patient; and
2. To protect the subject health-care provider from potential legal entanglements that may result from a patient's injury or death resulting as a consequence during the intra- or post-op procedure.

A legally signed consent form must be signed by the patient or a legally designated family member before the subject procedure can take place.

General Requirements for Informed Consent

The following items are required to be included in a consent form: the nature of the procedure, the risks and benefits [of] the procedure, reasonable alternatives, risks and benefits of alternatives, and assessment of the patient's understanding of the first four elements.[433]

"Patient Beware!"

I will take this opportunity to strongly advise you, the reader, or a family member to not just automatically sign a consent form, as typically is done during a closing for a house purchase, before any surgical procedure, especially if the procedure involves potential risks, as most do.

Many patients and their family members believe that the consent form is a mere formality and requires little, if any, scrutiny or review.

---

[433] Guide to Medical Device Regulations, Food and Drug Administration (FDA), Department of Health and Human Services. Part 50 – Protection of Human Subjects. No Date. Subpart A – General Provisions. Appendix II.

Quite the contrary. Thus, they blindly sign a document that may involve life-and-death decisions, fully trusting the integrity of its contents. In many of the hundreds of cases I have investigated, very bad decisions were made by patients who were not fully informed to the extent required under FDA regulations and law.

Those responsible for producing the contents of the consent form are required by law (the FD&C Act) and applicable FDA regulations to provide full disclosure within their consent form involving all surgical procedures.

Full Disclosure

The term *full disclosure* can be defined as the identification of all reasonably foreseeable information that could increase the probability of a safer and more effective procedure or device performance and/ or the identification of potential risks and hazards associated with the procedure or device used to reduce the risk through product and procedure labeling, including the consent form.

Pertaining to the use of any medical products, the primary objective and regulatory obligation of the product manufacturer is to include within the product labeling full disclosure by communicating to the fullest reasonable extent what must be accomplished for the product to be used in a safe, effective, and reliable manner, in response to its design objective intent and in accordance with its prescribed and authorized use by the FDA.

Therefore, when the appropriate health-care provider receives a new medical product to be used during a surgical procedure, they must extract from the manufacturer's labeling all applicable information specific to any and all potential risks and hazards that could occur during its intended use. This, of course, assumes the manufacturer has accomplished full disclosure within their product labeling, which I have discovered on many case investigations they did not. Typically physicians and other health-care providers do not read the manufacturer's labeling for the subject medical device or hospital equipment. This concern is particularly problematic if the device manufacturer changed the labeling involving new potential risks or hazards.

If the device manufacturer has not accomplished full disclosure within their device labeling, then the FDA would deem the device to be misbranded, and thus it could not be legally used, especially pertaining to a surgical procedure. Nor can the device be released into commercial distribution.

During my investigation of many hundreds of medical products involved with patient injuries and deaths, I have determined that a large percentage of the involved medical products were ultimately deemed to be misbranded. As such, these devices were illegally released and should not have been available to the hospital or the surgeons for use.

Warning for You and Your Family

It is imperative that individuals presented with a consent form by their health-care provider take the time and make the effort to fully comprehend the contents of the consent form before they agree to proceed with any surgical procedure.

Making every effort to being fully informed about all the critical details that should be evaluated and considered by the patient and/or their legally designated family member or other vested individuals is critical and may prove to be lifesaving.

On many occasions, I have had patients or family members inform me that had they been previously informed of the potential risks or hazards associated with the subject procedure made known to them, they or their family member would most likely not have elected to go forward with the procedure that resulted in a serious injury or the death of the patient.

Many of the cases I investigated involved patients who did not recognize the significance of the risks identified in the consent form they signed, resulting in the patient suffering a serious injury or death, and on some occasions, the known hazards and risks were not previously disclosed in their patient consent form.

Until an appropriate consent form containing full disclosure details is presented to the patient or designated family member for review and signature, any surgical procedure, especially a procedure deemed to involve a critical medical device, should be stopped dead in its tracks.

How to Determine If You Received Full Disclosure

Most individuals simply do not appreciate what issues must be addressed in their review of the consent form, in order to be assured that they have been fully informed of all applicable risks and other significant concerns.

Many patients simply sign consent forms even when they are anticipating a serious surgical procedure that could result in a serious injury or even death, without having an appropriate understanding of the risks and hazards involved with their forthcoming surgical procedure.

To assist you with your potential future review of a consent form and a determination if indeed you have been fully informed, I offer the following, although in certain circumstances other issues may go beyond these considerations. Nonetheless, the following discussion is indeed applicable to the vast majority of cases involving anticipated surgical procedures.

You may find it difficult to ask your health-care provider or your physician some of the direct questions pertaining to the key issues discussed below. Most patients and family members feel somewhat reluctant to question their doctor because they fear how their doctor may interpret question(s) such as inferring doubt in their capability to safely and effectively perform the procedure. Many times, the patient and their family members develop perceived friendships with their physician, especially when they have had many office visits or meetings with their doctor.

Most physicians will automatically provide some basic pre-surgical insights about the procedure and the anticipated post-surgical follow-up, but they seldom will address more detailed or specific insights related to many other aspects presented within the consent form, or even absent from the consent form, which is even a bigger concern.

While the patient's intent is certainly not to offend the health-care provider, it is imperative that the patient formulate a more inquisitive attitude in order to bridge any hesitation that would hinder being fully informed about the pending procedure and follow-up issues.

I have learned from discussions with many post-op patients who subsequently suffered a serious injury associated with the surgical procedure or the family members of patients who died during or shortly after their surgical procedure that they were never informed, in any manner, of the circumstance that either contributed to or directly caused the patient's serious injury or death.

This is not to infer in any manner that the physician has purposed to withhold vital information from the patient. Rather, they simply believe they have an adequate understanding of the following topics and do not believe it is necessary to pass so many details onto the patient or their family members unless such related questions are asked.

Therefore, it is my strong recommendation that every effort should be made to assure that full disclosure is presented within the consent form relevant to the subject surgical procedure before making a decision to proceed or not to proceed by the patient or family members.

Prior to your visit with your surgeon, discuss with your family and/or other concerned individuals the contents of your consent form. Identify any potential concerns and questions you want to discuss with your surgeon. Even if your consent form accomplished full disclosure, there may be terminology that is unfamiliar to you. Your goal is to fully comprehend and understand the contents of the consent form. This will, at minimum, give you greater peace of mind.

The time spent visiting with the surgeon (prior to the procedure) is important to assure that all such concerns are addressed. I recommend that the patient and/or family members specifically ask the surgeon, "Are all the potential risks and hazards associated with the procedure identified within the consent form?" or "Are there any concerns about the procedure you have that are not identified within the consent form?" If any subsequent injuries were to occur or even unexpected death, having presented your concerns as recommended above, it will prove particularly significant should it become appropriate to proceed with legal action.

I realize your thoughts might tend to blow off my recommendations, or you may believe your physician has become your friend. However, I base my recommendations on thirty-five years of forensic experience, academic study, and research.

Pre-Surgical Recommendations

First, review this list and ask any questions you or your family members may require for a greater understanding and record your questions under each main heading. Of course, there may be some items that you may not believe any further insights are required; however, I recommend you discuss each item with your family members in order to assure that there are no questions from all involved.

1. Intended Use: Ask what specific devices and equipment will be used during the procedure and what risks and hazards are associated with each.
2. Directions for Use: This is potentially a critical issue. Ask if the health-care provider performing the procedure is following the manufacturer's directions for use or if the physician intends to go off-label. If the physician has forethought or an expectation to use a medical product for purposes not presented within the context of the device labeling,

the physician must fully inform the patient and/or family members before the procedure about their anticipated use of the device, including issues associated with the off-label use, including the ramifications in terms of lack of evidence to support the safety, efficacy, and increased risk associated with such use.

3. Contraindications: This must identify all reasonably foreseeable situations where the surgical application or use of the device(s) may present a hazard to the patient. The use of any medical device or hospital equipment involving areas contraindicated in the product or equipment labeling, represents a serious departure from FDA-approved labeling and negligent off-label use.

4. Warnings: These are significant precautionary statements to the user indicating reasonably foreseeable uses whereby the user and/or the patient could be subjected to a hazardous event. Warnings advise the user of dangers that may occur if the instructions for its safe use are disregarded or the product is used improperly.

5. Precautions: This can be as vital as a warning. Precautionary statements attempt to protect the patient against the use of a device in such a manner that may result in device failure, injury, or death. Precautions typically focus on procedural concerns identified by the manufacturer where particular care must be exercised to avoid a device failure or hazard associated with the use of the device prescribed by the treating physician.

6. Adverse Effects: These describe potentially negative consequences that may result from use of the device, even if such use is in full compliance with its labeling contents.

Any omission of a reasonably foreseeable adverse effect not presented in the labeling (and subsequently the consent form) denies the patient an opportunity to make a fully informed decision as to whether they should consent to the procedure.

These recommendations are primarily intended for serious, potential life-threatening surgical procedures. While you may perceive that these recommendations are not necessary for you or your family confidence for a successful surgical outcome, I can assure you seeking as much pre-surgical details as possible may prove to be particularly advantageous if an adverse event should occur during or after the procedure.

As a medical forensic examiner, I have witnessed many cases that resulted in a serious injury to the patient and even death during a surgical procedure that resulted in an off-label application, failure of the device, or caused by the physician or other health-care provider.

In my own family, my father died at age fifty-five while in recovery from a surgical procedure when he went into shock from internal blood loss. To this day, I remain highly suspect that a surgeon's failure was directly the cause of my father's death. However, at the time, I was too young and years away from becoming a qualified forensic examiner to investigate the matter.

When I initially investigate a case involving a patient who has been seriously injured or died during or after a surgical procedure, I am required to consider all aspects of the proverbial causation pie. For example, all possible contributing eventualities must be thoroughly investigated in attempting to determine what aspect of each potential causation factor may have caused or contributed, in part or whole, to the patient's serious injury or death.

The specific areas of concern involve, for the most part, the following: user error [all health-care providers who participated during the surgical procedure (e.g., physicians, nurses, etc.)]; the device or drug manufacturer; improper or inadequate design; labeling; the patient; the health-care facility (hospital, clinic, etc.); outside participants (e.g., manufacturer representatives who participated during the surgical procedure); post-op care; and any other potential incidental contributing factors.

Often my final conclusions will indicate that a single causation factor resulted in the patient's serious injury or death, but not always. Sometimes two or more causation factors can be identified as responsible for the patient's serious injury or death, however, usually at different levels of accountability.

Acceptance Criteria

In addition to the tangible aspects associated in deciding whether to proceed with a potential surgical procedure, two other primary areas influence the decision-making process. These include our views on any related bioethical or medical ethics concerns and implications associated with our religious beliefs, if applicable.

These decision-making criteria are an inherent part of our being, formulated through our life experience, and constitute the unique characteristics of who we are. Our individual perspectives, especially pertaining to highly controversial issues, are unique to the individual because no two individuals retain the exact same life experiences.

Usually when we make a decision involving right or wrong or whether to support a certain cause or not, we chose a direction without specifically focusing on our inherent ethical or religious beliefs. In other words, as we experience issues during the evolution of our progressive life, we inherently and subconsciously mold and modify our attitude regarding these critical and even not-so-critical issues based on our interpretation of a positive or negative experience associated with the event.

The dramatic observations we witness every day in the newspaper and on TV bear witness to the strong and opposing opinions and views help by our political decision-makers, protesters, and other strongly opinionated people. Bring up any of the more controversial subjects (e.g., politics, gun control, birth control, immigration, environment, race relations, police, etc.), and the individual perspective will cover a broad spectrum of opinions, for and against. Moreover, even if a group supported one side of an ethical or religious issue, individuals would assign a different value to the subject issue.

Some individuals hold such strong and unwavering opinions pertaining to some of the more controversial subjects, like politics, for example, that they have severed ties with their opposing friends and family members. You can test this ethical or religious phenomenon with your family and friends. However, be careful not to push too hard to avoid jeopardizing relationships. Pick any controversial topic and ask each participant their opinion on the subject. You may already recognize that certain controversial topics are off-limits for discussion with certain family members. Then open up the matter for discussion. You will most likely note that some family members or friends will tend not to relinquish their opinion or perspective, no matter how significant the opposing and counter opinions support and justify an opposing opinion. You may also note that the stronger the opposition to a particular topic becomes, the stronger the defense for holding onto the individual's original position becomes.

Synergism is extremely difficult to accomplish when controversial subjects are involved. When was the last time during a heated discussion with someone that you heard them say, "Gee, you're right. I didn't think about that perspective."? I suspect it has been a long time, if ever. It's simply our human nature to hold onto our opinions, especially if the discussion becomes more heated. Our tendency would become even more entrenched and defensive. At a certain point in the discussion, now turned into an argument, any possibility of a synergetic outcome is now not possible, and to protect the future relationship of the debating individuals, the discussion should end.

25

DNA Damage Theory

The DNA damage theory of aging proposes that aging is a consequence of unrepaired accumulation of naturally occurring DNA damage. Damage in this context is a DNA alteration that has an abnormal structure. Several review articles have shown that deficient DNA repair, allowing greater accumulation of DNA damages, causes premature aging and that increased DNA repair facilitates can provide greater longevity.[434]

Freitas and de Magalhaes presented a comprehensive review and appraisal of the DNA damage theory of aging, including a detailed analysis of many forms of evidence linking DNA damage to aging. As an example, they described a study showing that centenarians of 100 to 107 years of age had higher levels of two DNA enzymes than the general population of older individuals of sixty-nine to seventy-five years of age.[435]

Their analysis supported the hypothesis that improved DNA repair leads to a longer life span. Overall, they concluded that while the complexity of responses to DNA damage remains only partly understood, the idea that DNA damage accumulation with age as the primary cause of aging remains an intuitive and powerful one.

---

[434] "DNA damage theory of aging," en.Wikipedia.org/wiki/DNA damage theory of aging.
[435] Id.

Nanotechnology

Nanomedicine is a future anticipated ability to repair damaged cells considered responsible for aging. K. Eric Drexler is one of the founders of nanotechnology who speculates that cell repair machines will operate within the cell using molecular computers to affect the repair.[436] In his book, *The Singularity Is Near,* Drexler states that advanced medical nanorobotics could **completely remedy the effects of aging** by 2030 (emphasis added).[437]

Although nanorobotics procedures may one day possibly provide a dramatic and exciting capability for life extension, it is doubtful that such technology would be fully developed by the year 2030. One major hurdle for the developer and research team involving nanorobotics is obtaining approval from the FDA for its intended use.

The time required to even approach the Agency with a proposal to proceed with clinical studies would require, as a prerequisite for FDA's permission to perform such studies, many years involving very stringent control and oversight by the FDA.

Moreover, assuming the FDA would permit the stakeholders to initiate clinical studies and assuming the clinical studies are completed and appropriate (in the mind of the sponsor) for submittal to the FDA with sufficient data to support formidable task of preparing the final submittal documents, referred to as Premarket Approval (PMA) submittal documents would undoubtedly involve many years beyond 2030, if approved at all.

Nonetheless, Ray Kurzweil, an American computer scientist and inventor who is currently the director of engineering for Google, believes that soon technology will give humankind the ability to place powerful machines in the human body to replace or improve existing biological systems.[438]

---

[436] "Life extension," en.wikipedia.org/wiki/Life extension.

[437] Id.

[438] R. Kurzweil, "To Count Our Days: The Scientific and Ethical Dimensions of Radical Life Extension," https://www.pewforum.org/2013/08/06/to-count-our-days-the-scientific-and-ethical-dimensions-of-radical-life-extension.

Kurzweil and other scientists believe that greater computing power combined with extreme miniaturization (nanotechnology) will allow scientists to put microscopic machines in the body, at first to protect and maintain people's organs and ultimately to effectively replace them. In essence, Kurzweil believes scientists will reverse-engineer bodily systems so they can be replaced with much more reliable machines.[439]

---

[439] Id.

26

The Human Organ

The human organ is defined as follows:

> An organ is a collection of tissues joined in a structural unit to serve a common function. Many organs are composed of a major tissue that performs the organ's main function, as well as other tissues that play supporting roles.[440]

The human body contains five primary organs vital for survival and include the following that work together to achieve a specific function:

- The brain controls thoughts, memory, and other organs.
- The heart pumps blood around the body.
- The kidneys filter blood and produce urine.
- The liver removes poisons from the blood.
- The lungs separate oxygen from the air and remove carbon dioxide from other main organs.
- The stomach helps to digest food.
- The intestines absorb nutrients from food.

---

[440] K. Kumar, "What Are the 78 Organs of the Human Body?" https://www.bbc.co.uk/bitesize/topics/znyycdm/articles/zbpdqhv.

- The bladder stores urine.
- The skin protects and contains the other organs.[441]

Seven non-vital body organs can be entirely removed without affecting a normal existence, including spleen, stomach, reproductive organs, colon, gallbladder, appendix, and kidneys.[442]

Transplanting Vital Organs

When a vital human organ can no longer perform its critical function effectively, many are capable of being replaced by removing a healthy organ from a human donor and surgically replacing the defective organ with the donor's organ.[443] This is a common occurrence that takes place almost every day.

Thus, through the replacement of defective vital organs with transplanted healthy organs from human donors, life extension and awareness are accomplished, while in the past these individuals would certainly have died.

Some scientists believe that in the foreseeable future, all body parts will be replaceable with enhanced components that could extend longevity and continued awareness. However, these same scientists do not believe that even if such capability did exist, it most likely would not become the standard mode for the purpose of extending length of life.[444]

However, Jean Hebert, PhD, believes that organs and tissues that

[441] Id.
[442] A. Taylor, "Seven body organs you can live without," https://theconversation.com/seven-body-organs-you-can-live-without-84984.
[443] "Organ Donation and Transplantation," https://my.clevelandclinic.org/health/articles/11750-0rgan-donation-and-transplantation.
[444] Replacing Body Parts," https://www.scientificamerican.com/article/replacing-body-parts/

come from donors are not a valid source for the treatment of aging individuals who are otherwise disease-free.[445]

Successful transplants of organs and tissues have included liver, kidney, pancreas, heart, lung, intestine, cornea, middle ear, skin, bone, heart valves, and other human body parts.[446]

There are more than 116,000 Americans on a waiting list who require an organ transplant, including about twenty who die each day while waiting for a donor.[447] However, even when an appropriate organ donor is presented, the cost for such dramatic transplants are quite formidable and not attainable for most individuals. For example, consider the following current average costs for transplantation procedures:

Estimated Cost for Procedure

Transplant	Cost
Double Lung	$1,397,000
Heart	$1,382,400
Intestinal transplant	$1,147,300
Bone marrow	$892,700
Lungs	$861,700
Liver	$812,500
Kidney	$414,800
Pancreas	$347,000
Cornea	$30,200[448]

[445] J. Herbert, "The Science of Replacement as a Means of Escaping Aging," blogs.einstein.yu.edu/the-science-of-replacement-as-a-means-of-escaping-aging.

[446] "Organ Donation and Transplantation," https://my.clevelandclinic.org/health/articles/11750-0rgan-donation-and-transplantation.

[447] N. Rapp, "Here's What Every Organ in the Body Would Cost to Transplant," https://fortune.com/2017/09/14/organ-transplant-cost/#:-:text=It's another thing to consider, transplant runs just over %24400%2C000.

[448] Id.

Insurance companies are reluctant to approve the more expensive transplants, not just for the surgical procedure but because of the post-surgical follow-up concerns as well.

Average Waiting Time for Organs

Organ	Waiting Time
Kidney	679 Days
Pancreas	281 Days
Liver	239 Days
Heart	191 Days
Lung	185 Days
Intestine	181 Days[449]

In 2021, more than 110,000 Americans were waiting for an organ transplant. Standing single file, that would form a line over fifty-two miles long. And that list is growing longer. Every ten minutes, someone is added to the transplant waiting list. That would equate to about 167 new candidates every day.

---

[449] Id.

27

Bionics and Prosthetic Devices

Bionics is defined as the technique of replacing a limb or body part like an artificial limb or part that is electronically or mechanically powered. Prosthetic is defined as an artificial device used to replace a missing body part, such as a limb, tooth, eye, or heart valve.[450]

Today, robotic assist prosthetic devices make it possible to duplicate the natural movement of the leg by using the person's mind. The user sends instructions from their brain, down through nerves that communicate with their mechanical limb. A new bionic arm powered by the thoughts of the user allows the person to deal cards, tie shoelaces, use a spoon, open drawers, and perform other hand movements; electronic legs allow paraplegics to walk upright. Today, bionic and prosthetic devices are available for almost every body part.[451]

---

[450] J. Williams, "Here Comes the Bionic Man: Disabled People Will Benefit," www.atechnews.com/newsanalysis/bionicman.html.

[451] G. Schofield et al., "When does a human being die?" https://doi.org/10.1093/qjmed/bcu239, p.3. https://academic.oup.com/qjmed/article/108/8/605/1549487.

Example of Future Life Extension Devices (Brain Stem Death)

In the UK, brain stem death is considered a standard definition of death. This unique definition of death states that death is determined only by the cessation of the brain stem, not including the whole brain.[452] Some scientists have stated that it is conceivable that one day researchers might invent an artificial brain stem that reproduces its functions and complex connection network and that doctors might be able to plug the patient into this just before their native one fails, just as we currently intubate patients and ventilate them if their respiratory system fails.[453]

Brain stem death is one of many definitions of how death is determined. As pertains to the UK definition, science has indicated the potential, if not the probability that life need not be terminated as a result of its failure. Thus, under this circumstance, the subject patient would extend their life (awareness) beyond what was previously determined to be their end of life.

Organs Grown in the Lab

In the more distant future, implantable laboratory-grown organs, such as hearts and other solid organs, will transcend human body part transplants. However, the scientists at Wake Forest Institute for Regenerative Medicine (WFIRM) are getting closer every day to reproducing and perfecting many of the tissues, blood vessels, and other organs of the human body.[454]

Touted as an international leader in translating scientific discovery into clinical therapies, the physicians and scientists at WFIRM at Wake Forest Baptist Center in Winston-Salem, North Carolina, are

---

[452] Id.

[453] Id.

[454] R. Jefferson, "Engineering Implantable, Laboratory-Grown Organs To Cure Disease," https://www.forbes.com/sites/robinseatonjefferson/2018/06/13/engineering-implantable-laboratory-grown-organs-to-cure-disease/?sh=4482cba57bcb.

developing organs and tissue for virtually every part of the human body as they attempt to engineer more than thirty different replacement tissues and organs and to develop healing cell therapies, all within the same goal, to cure rather than just treat disease.[455] Dr. Anthony Atala, director, said that one of the solid organs the WFIRM team is working hard on today is the kidney. The organ that there is the most need for in transplantation is the kidney, he said. Eighty percent of people on the organ donor list are waiting for a kidney.[456]

More than three hundred scientists in the field of biomedical and chemical engineering, cell and molecular biology, biochemistry, pharmacology, physiology, materials science, nanotechnology, genomics, surgery, medicine, and others are working to translate the science of regenerative medicine into clinical therapies.[457]

Here again is another current and future scientific endeavor that will further extend the life of individuals with defective body parts who are currently waiting for a much-needed body part transplant. In the future, these individuals who wait in agony for an organ replacement, many of whom will die during their wait, will be able to receive a manufactured organ that will effectively replace and function as the original organ was intended to perform.

What Constitutes a Person?

Let's consider the natural human body without any changes, modifications, or additions, as was the condition not so many decades ago. However, as science and industry began providing more and more human body replacement parts, the original construction of the human body as formed at birth has given way to a large variety of artificial body components. This is especially the case involving implantable orthopedic devices like hips, knees, ankles, elbows, fingers, shoulders, and wrist joints. In addition, there is a variety of

---

[455] Id.

[456] Id.

[457] Id.

implantable spinal fixation devices, such as screws, plates, rods, and other miscellaneous spinal hardware.

With the increasing number of artificial devices being implanted every year, a larger portion of the human anatomy no longer represents the body parts originally provided at birth. Nonetheless, the definition of a human and their continued existence goes on without any apparent recognition of this obvious reality. No matter how many body parts are replaced, these individuals still remain defined as humans.

Scientists, researchers, and bio-engineers are nearing a time when all body parts will be replaceable. In the near and more distant future, the same will also be true for all body organs and any other remaining aspects of the human body. The only human organ that cannot be replaced, at least based on current scientific thinking, will be the human brain, not to say that the continued function of the brain will not be replaced, as it will.

So let's take this discussion to the extreme end of the spectrum regarding replaceable body parts including vital organs. Let's say, hypothetically, that a human in the future had every possible body part replaced except for the brain. Would such an individual still be considered a human person or described as some other type of human or non-human entity? Would you consider this individual to be a living person if its entire body construction and function, minus the brain, were artificial?

Many would argue that as long as a fully functional brain exists, then this entity would be considered a person. However, if every human body part below the neck was replaced and there was no remaining live tissue, would you still refer to this entity as a person? We are not talking about life here but rather what defines a human.

You Have Already Been Replaced

As with most things in life that require periodic maintenance and replacement of damaged or worn-out parts, so too does the human body. For example, to achieve maximum life extension in humans and reduce the damage caused by the aging process would require, when circumstances indicate the necessity, the replacement of damaged tissues, molecular repair or rejuvenation of deteriorated cells and tissue, and the reversal of harmful epigenetic (e.g., the development of an organism changes),[458] which is defined as the development of an organism from an undifferentiated cell, consisting in the successive formation and development of organs and parts that do not preexist in the fertilized egg.[459]

Dr. Robert Langer, professor of chemical and biomedical engineering at MIT and a pioneer of tissue engineering, has said, "I have not come across a part of the body that someone somewhere isn't working on." He also stated, "Someday every part [of the human body] will be replaceable, even if that day is centuries away."[460]

Other scientists believe, as do I, that all parts of the human body will ultimately be replaceable and much sooner based upon the accelerated rate of accomplishments in all relevant areas of medicine and research as inhibiting obstacles are overcome. There is, however, in my opinion and many other scientists, one exception to replacing all human body parts, the brain. Nor would there be any reason to do so because there should be other future methods of assuring that human awareness can continue, as discussed in chapter 21.

Replacing Other Body Parts

If not yourself, most of us know someone who has received a medical device implant. With each passing year, medical scientists and engineers are developing more medical devices, cleared and approved by the FDA for release into commercial distribution that either extends the patient's life, addresses pain, or replaces a defective

---

[458] "Epigenetic," Medical Dictionary, 27th ed.
[459] "Life extension," en.wikipedia.org/wiki/Life extension.
[460] L. Villarosal, "How Much Of the Body Is Replaceable?" https://www.nytimes.com/2003/11/11/science/how-much-of-the-body-is-replaceable.html.

or damage body component for a higher quality of life. For example, consider the following partial list of medical devices identified under their appropriate category, currently available to patients, most involving implantable devices. There are many other medical devices not listed.

Cardiovascular Devices

- Vascular embolization device
- Cardiovascular intravascular filter
- Ventricular bypass (assist) device
- External and implantable pacemakers
- Cardiovascular electrodes
- Carotid sinus nerve stimulator
- Heart valves[461]

General and Plastic Surgery Devices

- Surgical mesh
- Breast prosthesis (two types)
- Chin prosthesis
- Esophageal prosthesis
- Nose prosthesis
- Tracheal prosthesis[462]

Neurological Devices

- Skull plate
- Carotid artery clamp
- Aneurysm clip
- Central nervous system fluid shunt
- Neuromuscular stimulator

---

[461] Code of Federal Regulations (CFR). Food and Drugs, Parts 800-1299. Revised April 1, 2017. Part 870 – Cardiovascular Devices.
[462] Id., Part 878 – General and Plastic Surgery Devices.

- Implanted cerebellar stimulator
- Implanted diaphragmatic nerve stimulator
- Implanted intracerebral stimulator (for pain)
- Implanted spinal cord stimulator (for pain)
- Implanted neuromuscular stimulator
- Implanted peripheral nerve stimulator (for pain)
- Transcutaneous electrical nerve stimulator (for pain)
- Dura substitute
- Electroconvulsive therapy device[463]

Obstetrical and Gynecological Devices

- Cervical drain
- Fallopian tube prosthesis
- Surgical mesh[464]

Ophthalmic Devices

- Artificial eye
- Eye sphere implant
- Intraocular lens[465]

Orthopedic Devices

- Bone cap
- Bone fixation cerclage
- Implanted intramedullary fixation rod
- Bone cement
- Implanted bone fixation device
- Spinal fixation device
- Implant pedicle screws
- Intervertebral body fusion device

---

[463] Id., Part 882 – Neurological Devices.
[464] Id., Part 884 – Obstetrical and Gynecological Devices.
[465] Id., Part 886 – Ophthalmic Devices.

- Implanted ankle joint (three types)
- Implanted elbow joint (four types)
- Implanted finger joint (four types)
- Implanted hip joint (fourteen types)
- Implanted knee joint (fourteen types)
- Implanted shoulder joint (six types)
- Implanted toe joint (two types)
- Wrist joint (seven types)[466]

The Eleven Most Implanted Medical Devices In America

Medical Device	Number of Yearly Procedures	Average Cost Per Procedure
1. Cardioverter Defibrillators	133,262	$40,000
2. Artificial Hips	230,000	$45,000
3. Heart Pacemakers	235,567	$20,000
4. Breast Implants	366,000	$3,351
5. Spinal Fusion Hardware	413,000	$25,000
6. Intra-Uterine Device (IUDs)	425,000	$800
7. Traumatic Fracture Repair	453,000	$2,000–$20,000
8. Artificial Knees	543,000	$22,000
9. Coronary Stents	560,000	$13,000
10. Ear Tubes	715,000	$1,000–$4,500
11. Artificial Eye Lenses	2,582,000	$3,200–$4,500[467]

Artificial Organ Implants

Another option for the replacement of defective organs involves artificial organs. An artificial organ is a human-made organ device or tissue that is implanted or integrated into a human, interfacing with living tissue, to replace a natural organ or to duplicate or augment a

---

[466] Id., Part 888 – Orthopedic Devices.

[467] Wall Street Business Insider, "The 11 Most Implantable Medical Devices In America," https://www.businessinsider.com/the-11-most-implanted-medical-devices-in-america-2011-7#11-implantable-cardioverter-defibrillators-icds-1.

specific function or functions so the patient may return to a normal life as soon as possible,[468] thereby extending the patient's life.

One significant disadvantage of an artificial organ as compared with a transplanted human organ is that the artificial organ may require many years of continued maintenance service.[469]

Examples of Artificial Implants

Artificial organs include prosthetic limbs (with robotic attachments), bladder, penile implants (two types), testes, ear (cochlear implant), eye (external miniature digital camera), heart (implantable heart valves, implantable pacemakers, implantable defibrillators, and implantable ventricular assist device), kidney (support device), lungs (pending near future development), extracorporeal membrane oxygenation (ECMO) (used to take significant load off the lung and heart),[470] extracorporeal CO_2 removal (ECCO2R) (benefits the patient through carbon dioxide removal rather than oxygenation, with the goal of allowing the lungs to relax and heal),[471] ovaries (pending future development), pancreas, thymus (pending future development), trachea (pending future development), implantable drug dispenser, and electrodes and wires.

Other Current Technologies Producing Body Replacement Parts

Following are ten existing technologies currently available to a patient to replace body parts that either improve the well-being of the patient or extends their life span:

1. 3D printed bones (printed replica of bone using titanium alloy)

---

[468] "Artificial Organ," en.wikipedia.org/wiki/Artificial organ.
[469] Id.
[470] Id.
[471] Id.

2. Chip implants (implanted in hand will enable person to open doors, log onto computers, etc. by waving hand)
3. Bioprinter organs (used to repair or replace damaged human organs)
4. Brain to computer (implant connects the brain to a computer using electrodes)
5. Replica nose (provides smelling without a real biological nose)
6. Enhanced immune system (adjusting the body's immune system)
7. Bionic eyes (provides sight to those who cannot see)
8. Cochlear implants (helps deaf people to hear)
9. Exoskeletons (wearable machines to improve limb performance of paraplegia or spinal cord injury patients, giving them the ability to walk again)
10. Designer babies[472]

One of the most controversial applications of technology to human bodies is designer babies. While some view embryo editing as dangerous and ethically abhorrent, new gene-editing techniques could be used to detect and prevent inherited diseases in fetuses. There is still a lot of debate to be had before the technique can be applied to embryos that develop into babies.[473]

While conducting research many years ago involving non-thrombogenic implantable materials at the University of Minnesota (e.g., for materials tending not to be rejected by the human body), I recognized that the human body often chooses to reject what it considers a foreign substance (e.g., any material not naturally produced by the human body itself). Scientists and engineers have continued to develop many biomedical materials and related adaptations now readily accepted by the body. These materials include titanium, silicone, ceramics, polyethylene, and others. Researchers and biomaterial engineers, for the most part, have finally overcome the body's tendency to reject foreign materials implanted within the body.

---

[472] Disruption Hub, "10 Technologies Replacing Your Body Now," August 29, 2017.
[473] Id.

28

The 15 Highest-Grossing Prescription Drugs in America (Based upon Gross Sales Volume)

Drug	Prescription Purpose
1. Lipitor	Used to reduce the risk of heart attack and stroke
2. Nexium	Used by patients with acid reflux to treat heartburn
3. Plavix	Used to prevent blood clots by patients at risk for strokes and heart attacks
4. Advair Diskus	Used to treat asthma symptoms
5. Abilify	Used to treat schizophrenia and bipolar disorders
6. Seroquel	Used to treat schizophrenia and bipolar disorders
7. Singulair	Used to treat asthma
8. Crestor	Used to reduce cholesterol
9. Actos	Used to treat type 2 diabetes
10. Epogen	Used by patients with chronic failure to treat anemia
11. Remicade	Used to treat Crohn's disease and rheumatoid arthritis
12. Enbrel	Used to treat inflammatory disease, including arthritis
13. Cymbalta	Used to treat depression and anxiety disorders
14. Avastin	Used by cancer patients as part of tumor-starving therapy.
15. Oxycontin	Used as a painkiller for moderate to severe pain[474]

---

[474] C. Jenkins, "The 15 Highest Grossing Prescription Drugs In America," https://www.businessinsider.com/highest-gross-prescription-drugs-2011-4#did-you-know-that-medical-bills-are-the-number-one-reason-for-bankruptc.

Dangers Associated with Prescription Drugs

Without question, the drugs that physicians prescribe to treat various ailments can and do extend our lives. When we describe our symptoms to the doctor, they will attempt to identify the most appropriate drug and dosage to hopefully elevate the symptoms and possibly cure the condition.

Some drugs prescribed are potentially dangerous if not taken exactly as prescribed or if they are inadvertently taken involving dangerous combinations with other drugs or alcohol. For example, the number of adults in the United States who experience pain (not due to cancer) rose from about 32 percent in 1998 to 41 percent in 2014, but the number of people taking opioid painkillers to deal with their pain doubled.

In keeping with this increase in painkiller use, the rate of people who have died from overdoses of prescription painkillers, including oxycodone (OxyContin), hydrocodone (Vicodin), and fentanyl, has increased massively over the past decade. In 2017, over 17,000 Americans died from taking prescribed painkillers.[475]

Here's a shocker for you: In a list of the top-ten most dangerous drugs, most people would not think of a drug as common as acetaminophen. However, according to 24/7 Wall Street's Investigation,[476] it shows that what we typically think of as "just Tylenol" can be considered the world's most dangerous drug. Acetaminophen is responsible for some of the most dangerous drug interactions. There is a high potential for toxicity and liver damage from an overdose of acetaminophen. Additionally, because most people view the drug as innocuous, that perception may contribute to its unintentional abuse.[477]

The reality that a common over-the-counter drug such as Tylenol

---

[475] E. Hartney, "Five Dangerous Classes of Prescription Drugs," https://www.verywellmind.com/most-deadly-prescription-drugs-4083005.

[476] https://247wallst.com/special-report/ 2019/07/25/25-mostdangerous-drugs-3/

[477] J. Youell, "The 25 Most Dangerous Drugs May Not Be What You Think," https://www.therecoveryvillage.com/drug-addiction.

being so potentially hazardous should caution us all to be particularly careful with the drugs we take. I am aware of a perverse attitude by many individuals who casually assume, *Well, since I still have a headache, I'll just take a few more pills.* Herein lies the potential hazard of overdosing oneself.

Very few individuals ever read the packaged insert labeling in order to determine the FDA's authorized labeling that describes, among other relevant and important details about the subject drug, the known side effects associated with taking the drug. I have investigated cases where patients have suffered serious injury and death resulting from not understanding, not being aware of, or ignoring the stated serious side effects presented within the drug (or device) labeling.

To clarify: The optimum effect of any drug (over-the-counter or especially prescription) is to target the envelope of maximum effective response (ideal dosage). For example, consider the following representation: potential toxicity (overdose), ideal dosage, and ineffective dosage. The prescribing physician will attempt, based upon their examination, test results, and prognosis of the patient's described ailment, the appropriate medication and dosage should remedy the ailment.

Physicians will most often tend to under-prescribe the dosage, particularly when potentially dangerous drugs are involved, and then readjust the dosage at a follow-up visit rather than risk the possibility of an overdose.

It is also important to clarify the issue of identified side effects associated with taking the subject medication. Notice the side effects described in TV commercials involving certain drugs advertised. It must frustrate the drug manufacturers who sell these drugs to be required under law to disclose the known side effects of the drug when they really want to only focus on the happy claims of taking their medication since they are aware that full disclosure requires them to inform the American public of the known hazards associated with the drug usage. I have often questioned why anyone would take that drug with such serious potential side effects.

The pharmaceutical industry is tasked with the federal-mandated and FDA-regulated obligation to formulate drugs that effectively and safely provide the optimum treatment for specific conditions and symptoms with the minimum side effects.

However, in order for any pharmaceutical manufacturer to effectively produce a drug that is in compliance with the applicable laws and regulations that govern what must be accomplished to persuade the FDA that the sponsor's drug will indeed provide the optimum medication, it will typically involve many years of continued dialogue with the Agency. Moreover, there is no guarantee that the sponsor-submitted new drug application will ever be approved.

More specific to the issue of side effects, the ultimate drug formulation must accept that certain identified side effects during their clinical investigation cannot be avoided. It boils down to accepting the reality that to design and formulate the optimum drug for the specific health ailment, certain negative side effects must be permitted. In other words, if attempts were made to reduce or eliminate the identified side effects, then the optimum medication must also be diminished in its effectiveness. Thus, the end result is to accomplish the maximum benefit with minimal risks (e.g., side effects).

Lastly, I recommend that you put a list of all the medications that you take in your wallet, including the prescribed dosage. Also, include any vitamins and aspirin (81 milligrams is popular) and any other supplements you are taking. This precaution could be a lifesaver, should you be involved in an accident, saving time for the health-care providers attempting to determine what medications you are currently taking. Keep the list updated.

Also, in addition to your prescribing physician, consider your pharmacist as a valuable resource of information about the drugs you are taking. They understand the uniqueness of the drug formulations and the associated dangers, including dangerous combination of certain drugs.

Therefore, the transplanting of vital tissue organs, or artificial organs, and the replacement of other body components, including the administration of current and future preventive and curative drugs, will continue to further defeat the aging process and extend life. Research and engineering efforts will continue each year to bring additional improvements in these areas to battle the relentless and inevitable encroachment of the aging process.

29

Living Will

If you do not have a living will, you may want to consider getting one. A living will is a written, legal document that spells out medical treatments you would and would not want to be used to keep you alive, as well as your preference for other medical decisions.

Assume it is your intent that at the time when your health may have deteriorated to near or at a critical stage of your continued existence, you desire to have the most advanced medical technology and drugs available to maintain your continued existence. Notice I did not infer awareness, which may or may not be a consideration for you dependent on your circumstances.

Without a living will, circumstances may arise where you are approaching the end of your life and are unable to voice your desire to have your existence prolonged by all available medical means. Perhaps you were aware of significant advances in medical research that could provide you with the possibility of having your life continued beyond your future death and wanted to survive long enough to take advantage of such medical advances.

Therefore, if it is your desire to take advantage of any medical technology or current and future advancements in medical treatment designed to extend your life, then you should assure that your wishes are fully and accurately described in a living will document.

Of course, the opposite desire to let life go should also be clearly indicated in the event your life is being maintained by artificial methods that are not acceptable to you.

30

Final Conclusions

This writing should have provided you with many significant insights to ponder about your life or the life of a loved family member, perhaps for the first time. Again, my attempt has been to consolidate a significant amount of relevant scientific data in order for you to develop a better understanding of the aging process and efforts underway to extend your life and your awareness.

My goal has been to ferret out from the enormous amount of diverse research material produced by many scientists in various areas of investigating the enigma that surrounds solutions to the aging process and extending human life in order to more effectively communicate this information to you.

This effort would have been far less formidable and less challenging if there were a more acceptable consensus of opinions among the scientists who have dedicated their careers to researching solutions to the aging process and extending human life.

Unfortunately, there were and remains strong and opposing opinions by these scientists on virtually every major issue involving both aging and life extension. Nonetheless, I believe I have been able to amalgamate the primary essence of where we currently reside and what the expectations are for the near and distant future pertaining to these two focused areas of discussion.

In a general sense, I have drawn a line in the sand where on one side the focus has involved all research activity, including currently available medical solutions, intended to extend your life and your awareness to the furthest extent within today's normal human life cycle.

On the other side of the line resides the current research that presents possible solutions and innovative thinking about how humanity may be able to extend human life and awareness beyond the end of the normal human life cycle.

The insights and speculations provided by these scientists have described various methods to accomplish the dramatic extension of human life and awareness beyond death indicates the possibility that one day humanity could conceivably continue to experience their further existence and awareness for many years, perhaps centuries beyond their human physical death.

The major areas of near and distant future discovery that will attempt to extend life discussed in this reading have included: brain transplant to a human body, brain transplant into a humanoid robot, body-to-head transplant (without the spinal cord), body-to-head transplant (with the spinal cord), AI and humanoid robots, human consciousness uploading/downloading, and implantable brain chips.

The issue of eternity as a possibility of continued human existence and awareness was also discussed involving those scientists who believe it can be achieved and those scientists (like myself) who do not believe that an eternal, immortal existence of awareness is possible.

However, if only for the sake of discussion, if there were indeed any remote possibility of an eternal, never-ending existence of awareness, and again I emphasize that in my opinion anything created by humanity cannot exist forever, then one absolute prerequisite would be the elimination of anything created by humanity as a necessity for the continued existence of that awareness.

In other words, an eternal existence must be totally absent of any substance that resides within the realm of humanity and the world. As long as there is any substance, no matter how small that would be involved with supporting a continued awareness and memories, then there cannot be any realistic expectation that under those circumstances, the subject awareness could exist forever. If there is any physical material or substance of any kind that exists and is required to enable the subject awareness to continue to exist, no matter for how long, the said substance will bind the awareness to the existing realm of humanity and thus prohibit any eternal existence.

To further clarify, in order to accomplish the implausible immortality I have alluded to previously, could only occur if the impossibility of maintaining a continued awareness with no physical relationship to an earthly substance was effective.

Not wanting to leave you wondering what I am referring to, let me expand just a little further. Two examples exist within the realm of nature and physics that could hypothetically play a part in the very distant future (although highly unlikely at any time in the foreseeable future) that could permit an awareness medium, for lack of a better word, to exist, yes, forever. One is sound; the other is light.

However, sound does not travel forever. Sound cannot travel through empty space; it is carried by vibrations in a material or medium (e.g., air, steel, water, wood, etc.). As the particles in the medium vibrate, energy is lost to heat, viscous (high resistance to flow) processes, and molecular motion. So the sound wave gets smaller and smaller until it disappears.[478]

Stay with me! In contrast, light waves can travel through a vacuum and do not require a medium, as does sound. In empty space, the wave does not dissipate (grow smaller), no matter how far it travels because the wave is not interacting with anything else. This is why light from distant stars and galaxies can travel through space for billions of light-years and still reach earth.[479]

Now, having said all that, let's imagine that in the distant future, scientists were actually able to convert human awareness into

---

[478] D. Schmid, "Does light [or sound] travel forever?" https://van.physics.illinois. edu/qa/listing.php?id=21368&t=does-light-travel-forever#:-:text=First%2C let's think about why,water%2Cwood%2Cetc).&t.
[479] Id.

something akin to a light beam and thereby transmit awareness within the context of the light beam into space since light beams would not be inhibited by the environment of space and not tethered to an earthly element.

I know this really sounds weird and purely destined for the sci-fi screen. However, even if this were possible, there remains a huge issue, mobility. How could a light beam traveling awareness possibly control or manipulate its location to an intended target location? It could not. At best, it may be able to be directed from its transmitter to some incredible receiver. Then what? Light can only travel in a straight line unless you want to consider some of Albert Einstein's thinking.

If by some inexplicable future discovery by scientists that developed a process by where they could actually control the direction and movement of light with its association to awareness, could there be, even under these circumstances, a remote possibility that human awareness could exist forever, true immortality? I think not! Well, enough of the science fiction because that's all immortality could ever be.

Nonetheless, I do believe based on, in part, much of the scientific discussion presented within this book that in the foreseeable, and especially within the more distant, future that humanity will achieve a continued existence and awareness for many years beyond our current comprehension.

While reading this book, I realize you were presented with some very dreadful predictions that may have caused you some disconcerting and perhaps fearful thoughts to ponder. I did consider not including those topics; however, since I believe that there is a significant and realistic possibility that such events may occur, I elected to include my conclusions and opinions on these topics for you to process. Knowledge and awareness are powerful cognitive tools and will separate those who possess them and know how to apply their benefits from the vast majority of the population, most of whom simply ramble through their daily existence without significant clarity or understanding beyond their daily concerns and endeavors.

Perhaps it was a mistake to do so; however, within the scientific world of research and discovery, I believe it is better not to stick our heads in the sand because we may not be able to face the reality of the inevitable. For example, if scientists were aware of an approaching meteorite of a size that would destroy the earth and the approximate time it would strike the earth, would you want to know or not?

Whatever your answer may be, consider why you made your decision and what your decision was based upon.

summary Thoughts

I sincerely hope that you found the contents of this book mentally stimulating with significant and serious issues to reflect upon. As there have been serious disagreements and opposing opinions between the scientists presented within the various topics relating to the aging process, life extension, immortality, awareness, and many related topics, I anticipate there would be those individuals who would agree with and those who would disagree with the positions I have taken regarding these same topics.

Underlining the overall content and controversy discussed within this book has been my intent to provide you with an unfettered discussion about issues seldom considered by those outside the scientific community, but are nonetheless particularly relevant to your continued existence.

One final thought (no pun intended) regarding awareness: The discussion on awareness also included an obvious appreciation of one's surroundings. However, awareness does not necessarily include adequate intelligence, certain areas of knowledge that would be relevant to our survival and well-being, or the ability to properly interpret and respond accordingly to the actual reality of one's surroundings, often due to lack of experience, knowledge, focus, or simply not caring.

For example, high school or college students who often have lived rather sheltered lives desire deeply to go on spring break to Florida, on a trip with friends to Europe, and so forth with considerable ignorance of the potential dangers that could befall them. Such potential hazards were clearly depicted in the movie *Taken*, starring Liam Neeson, where his daughter, not being completely honest with her father, travels with a friend to Europe and succumbs to the nefarious invitation of a stranger at the airport to share a cab ride and later to join him at a party. They are subsequently kidnapped until rescued by their father.

So much for youthful and sometimes vulnerable thinking. No one beyond their teen years, and perhaps younger, has not experienced making a bad decision based on their decision-making capability and experience at the time. We all retain some level of regret for past inappropriate decision-making and perhaps certain indiscretion. Such awareness of our past should emphasize our need to focus more effectively on our life experiences and thus develop a more focused awareness about our awareness.

Finally, as Spock always said on *Star Trek*, "Live long and prosper!"

Epilogue

During the evolution of this book, many hundreds of books, articles, journals, government documents, and legal records were carefully reviewed and scrutinized to collect the most relevant and succinct information and data to accomplish the primary objective of its targeted focus and readers.

Again, that objective was to approach a very complicated and highly controversial subject pertaining to the further extension of human life and especially human awareness and to translate its varied meanings into terminology that would prove interesting, insightful, stimulating, and even challenging to the reader.

There were occasions when I hesitated to include certain subjects due to the graphic and traumatic nature involved; however, I decided it was essential, and in keeping with a broader spectrum of issues related to human life extension, I decided to express these opinions involving some very troubling and prodigious anticipated future realities.

I assure you I did not include these catastrophic conclusions without adequate justification to support such dire anticipations of these probable future events. Of course, there will be many who challenge my dismal opinions; however, the factual realities and basic math are there for anyone interested enough to perform their own independent analysis. I encourage you to do so!

I certainly want to thank the hundreds of professional and scientific research individuals who published incredible insights into a realm of knowledge and pursuit seldom understood by those not involved in such areas of study. Their documented material provided substantial information and data for the creation of this book.

Although there were serious and significant disagreements between the many scientists pertaining to almost every key topic discussed, their varied opinions have nonetheless contributed to the further advancement of science and medicine for the greater good of humanity.

I have attempted to provide adequate and appropriate recognition within the citations for everyone who has provided specific insights presented throughout this book. As apparent by the many citations identified herein, I may have inadvertently failed to recognize all professional contributors. Should you recognize some aspect of your work not properly cited within this book, please accept my apologies and identify your valued contribution with hopes that you will continue to advance all aspects of your expertise to further extend the boundaries of human life and awareness.

Bibliography

Alban, D. "72 Amazing Human Brain Facts (Based on the Latest Science)." Last modified September 21, 2022. bebrainfit.com/human-brain-facts.

Aleksandrov, Y. 2017. "Between life and death: how to freeze yourself and wake up in future." https://medium.com/cryogen/between-life-and-death-how-to-freeze-yourself-and-wake-up-in-future-1ff8715abf80.

Andrade, G. n.d. "Immortality." https://iep.utm.edu>immortality.

Beckman, K. 2016. "9 Factors That Affect Longevity." https://www.thinkadvisor.com/2016/05/27/9-factors-that-affext-longevity.

Berger, T. 2013. "No Science Fiction: A Brain In A Box To Let People Live On After Death." https://www.fastcompany.com/3015553/not-science-fiction-a-brain-in-a-box-to-let-people-live-on-after-death.

Bhat, S. 2018. "Except for the brain, which organ cannot be transplanted?" https://www.quora.com/Except-for-the-brain-which-organ-cannot-be-transplanted.

Booth, F. 2011. "Lifetime sedentary living accelerates some aspects of secondary aging." https://journals.physiology.org/doi/full/10.1152/japplphysiol.00420.2011.

Calbernone, J. 2017. "Is Decaffeinated Coffee Bad for You?" https://www.consumerreports.org/coffee/is-decaffeinated-coffee-bad-for-you.

Cherry, K. 2020. "The Size of the Human Brain Medically Reviewed by Steven Gans, MD." https://www.verywellmind.com/how-big-is-the-brain-2794888#:-:text=manyother mammals.

Cohut, M. 2018. "Seven (or more) things you didn't know about your brain." https://www.medicalnewstoday.com/articles/322081#7.-Is-perception-a-controlled-hallucination?

Collins, L. 2013. "Radical life extension: What would you think of living to 120 and beyond, survey asks." htpps://www.deseret.com/2013/8/6/20523581/radical-life-extension-what-would-you-thinkof-living-to-120-and-beyond-survey-asks#maxine-t-grimm-ag.

Daley, J. 2019. "New Study Shows Coffee-Even 25 Cups a Day of It-Isn't Bad for Your Heart." https://www.smithsonianmag.com/smart-news/new-study-shows-coffee-even-25-cups-day-isnt-bad-for-heart-180972336/#:-:text=David DiSalvo at For.

Dance, A. 2017. "Scientists Want to Use Brain Implants to Tune the Mind." https://www.kavlifoundation.org/science-spotlights/scientists-want-use-brain-implants-tune-mind#.XxoEWJ5Kjcs.

de Grey, A. 2013. "To Count Our Days: The Scientific and Ethical Dimension of Radical Life Extension." In "Who Wants to Live Forever? Scientist sees aging cured." http://www.reuters.com/article/2011/07/04/us-aging:cure-idUSTRE76321D20110704.

Drew, L. 2019. "The ethics of brain – computer interfaces." https://www.nature.com/articles/d41586-019-02214-2.

Eschmann, B. n.d. "Is it scientifically possible to remove a human brain and place it in a robotic body, with most sensory capabilities?" https://www.quora.com/Is-it-scientifically-possible-to-remove-a-human-brain-and-place-it-in-a-robotic-body-with-most-sensory capabilities.

Fifield, K. 2020. "Dementia vs. Alzheimer's: Which Is It?" https://www.aarp.org/health/dementia/info-2018/difference-between-dementia-alzheimers.

Ford, D. 2011. "How the Brain Learns." *Training Industry*.

Frances, A. 2016. "A Debate on the Pros and Cons of Aging and Death." https://www.psychologytoday.com/us/blog/saving-normal/201612/debate-the-pros-and-cons-aging-and-death.

Furr, A. 2018. "Surgical, ethical, and psychosocial considerations in human head transplantation." https://www.sciencedirect.com/science/article/pii/S1743919117300808#:-:tex=Surgical%2C and psychosocial considerations in human.

Gkasdaris, G. 2019. "First Human Head Transplantation: Surgically Challenging, Ethically Controversial and Historically Tempting - an Experimental Endeavor or a Scientific Landmark?" https://www.ncbi.nlm.nih.gov/pmc/articles/PMC6511668.

Gnum, A. n.d. "If a brain transplant was successful, would the recipient think and act like the donor did?" https://www/quora.com/

If-a-brain-transplant-was-successful-would-the-recipient-think-and-act-like-the-donor did?

Gold, G. 2015. "This Is the Age When You Start to Visibly Look Older." https://www.marieclaire.com/beauty/news/a16636/the-age-when-aging-begins.

Graziano, M. 2019. "Will Your Uploaded Mind Still Be You?" https://www.wsj.com/articles/will-your-uploaded-mind-still-be-you-11568386410?mod=article_inline.

Gregory, A. 2019. "First human head transplant could be achieved by 2030, veteran NHS neurosurgeon claims." https://www.independent.co.uk/news/science/human-head-transplant-spinal-cord-nhs-chrysalis-bruce-matthew-canavero-neurosurgeon-a9256841.html.

Guzder, D. 2009. "When Parents Call God Instead of the Doctor." content.time.com/time/national/article/0,8599,1877352, 00.html.

Hanson Robotics. n.d. "Sophia. Connecting with humans." https://www.hansonrobotics.com/sophia.

Hartney, E. 2021. "Five Dangerous Classes of Prescription Drugs." https://www.verywellmind.com/most-deadly-prescription-drugs-4083005.

Hayward, J. "Fascinating Things About the Brain." Last modified February 21, 2020. https://www.activebeat.com/your-health/9-fascinating-things-about-the-brain/?utm_medium=cpc&utm_source=google_search_network&utmcampaign.

Herbert, J. 2018. "The Science of Replacement as a Means of Escaping Aging." blogs.einstein.yu.edu/the-science-of-replacement-as-a-means-of-escaping-aging.

Hulsroj, P. 2015. "What Is Immortality?" In *What If We Don't Die?*, 63–94. Springer Praxis Books.

Inafuku, J. 2010. "Downloading Consciousness." https://cs.stanford.edu/people/eroberts/cs181/projects/2010-11/DownloadingConsciousness/tandr.html.

Jackson, A. 2016. "The problem with human head transplants." https://theconversation.com/the-problem-with-human-head-transplants-535222.

Jefferson, R. 2018. "Engineering Implantable, Laboratory-Grown Organs To Cure Disease." https://www.forbes.com/sites/robinseatonjefferson/2018/06/13/engineering-implantable-laboratory-grown-organs-to-cure-disease/?sh=4482cba57bcb.

Jenkins, C. 2011. "The 15 Highest Grossing Prescription Drugs In America." https://www.businessinsider.com/highest-gross-prescription-drugs-

2011-4#did-you-know-that-medical-bills-are-the-number-one-reason-for-bankruptc.

Jennings, A. 2018. "Telepathy Is Real." https://www.facebook.com/Inside Science, p.2. https://insidescience.org/video/telepathy-real.

Jensen, K. 2020. "Will We Ever Be Able to Upload Our Brains?" https://www.pcmag.com/news/will-we-ever-be-able-to-upload-our-brains.

Johnson, R. 2018. "A review of vagus nerve stimulation as a therapeutic intervention." Doi:10.2147/JIR.S163248.

Jovanovic, T. n.d. "What is Anxiety?" https://www.anxiety.org/what-is-anxiety.

Juang, M. 2017. "Advances in brain pacemaker reduces tremors, helps Parkinson's sufferers live a more normal life." https://www.cnbc.com/2017/10/05/brain-pacemaker-stops-tremors-helps-parkinsons-sufferers.html.

Kochanek, M. 2019. "Leading Causes of Death, Centers for Disease Control and Prevention." In *Mortality in the United States*. NCHS Data Brief No. 395.

Kumar, K. 2021. "What Are the 78 Organs of the Human Body?" https://www.bbc.co.uk/bitesize/topics/znyycdm/articles/zbpdqhv.

Kurzweil, R. 2013. "To Count Our Days: The Scientific and Ethical Dimensions of Radical Life Extension." https://www.pewforum.org/2013/08/06/to-count-our-days-the-scientific-and-ethical-dimensions-of-radical-life-extension.

Lau, B. 2017. "10 most important medicines in history." MIMS Today.

Lee, J. n.d. "If a brain transplant was possible, what information would the transplanted brain retain in its new body?" https://www.quora.com/If-a-brain-transplant-was-possible-what-information-would-the-transplanted-brain-retain-in-its-new-body.

Lewis, T. 2021. "Human Brains: Facts, Functions & Anatomy." Live Science, p.2. https://www.livescience.com/29365-human-brain.html.

Maedica. 2019. "First Human Head Transplantation: Surgically Challenging, Ethically Controversial and Historically Tempting – an Experimental Endeavor or a Scientific Landmark?" https://www.ncbi.nlm.nih.gov/pmc/articles/PMC6511668.

Mailonline, H. 2018. "Pig brains are kept alive OUTSIDE their bodies for the first time in a radical experiment that could allow humans to become immortal." https://www.dailymail.co.uk/sciencetech/article-5659235/Pig-brains-kept-alive-WITHOUT-body-time.html.

Marr, B. 2020. "Artificial Human Beings: The Amazing Examples Of Robotic Humanoids And Digital Humans." https://www.forbes.com/

sites/bernardmarr/2020/02/17/artificial-human-beings-the-amazing-examples-of-robotic-humanoids-and-digital-humans/?sh=2.

Masci, M. 2015. "To Count Our Days: The Scientific and Ethical Dimensions of Radical Life Extension." https://www.pewresearch.org/experts/david-masci.

McGee, E. 2019. "Ethical Assessment of Implantable Brain Chips." https://www.bu.edu/wcp/Papers/Bioe/BioeMcGe.htm.

Melinosky, C. 2019. "Memory Loss." https://www.webmdcom/brain/memory-loss#1-2.

Mercadante, A. 2020. "Neuroanatomy, Gray Matter." Stat Pearls Publishing.

Miceli, C. 2018. "I Think Therefore I Am: Descartes on the Foundations of Knowledge." *Word Philosophy – An Introductory Anthology.*

Murali, J. 2019. "Immortality through mind uploading." https://www.deccanchronicle.com/opinion/op-ed/220719/immortality-through-mind-uploading.html.

Newan, T. 2017. "All you need to know about neurons." https://www.medicalnewstoday.com/articles/320289.

Novella, S. 2018. "Keeping Brains Alive Outside the Body." https://www.theness.com/neurologicablog/index.php/keeping-brains-alive-outside-the-body.

Olshansky, S. 2002. "Position Statement on Human Aging." https://academic.oup.com/biomedgerontology/article/57/8/B292/556758.

Paddock, C. 2018. "These five habits will lengthen your lifespan." https://www.medicalnewstoday.com/articles/321671#Life-expectancy-rises-with-each-factor.

Parson, J. 2020. "Futurologist claims super rich will 'live forever' by implanting brains into robots." https://metro.co.uk/futurologist-claims-super-rich-will-live-forever-implanting-brains-robots-12352856.

Parthasarathy, K. n.d. "Could we transplant our brains into robot bodies in order to gain immortality?" https://www.quors.com/Could-we-transplant-our-brains-into-robot-bodies-in-order-t-gain-immortality.

Peters, B. 2020. "What to Expect From a Head Transplant." https:/www.verywellhealth.com/head-transplant-4801452.

Pettit, H. 2018. "First human frozen by cryogenics could be brought back to life 'in just TEN years', claims expert. Daily Mail online." https://www.dailymail.co.uk/sciencetech/article-5270257/Cryogenics-corpses-brought-10-years.html.

Pietrangelo, A. "The Effects of Alcohol on Your Body." Last modified on September 28, 2018. https://www.healthline.com/health/alcohol/effects-on-body#4.

Pultarova, T. 2017. "Why Human Head Transplants Will Never Work." https://www.livescience.com/60987-human-head-transplants-will-never-work.html.

O'Neil-Pirozzi, T. n.d. "Traumatic Brain Injury Resource for Survivors and Caregivers." https://bouve.northeastern.edu/nutraumaticbraininjurybi-anatomy/brain-changes-over-the-lifespan.

Orrange, S. 2018. "8 Surprising Benefits of Metformin Besides Treating Diabetes." Good Rx, Inc.

Paavola, A. 2019. "10 most prescribed drugs in the U.S. in Q1." https://www.bechershospitalreview.com/pharmacy/10-most-prescribed-drugs-in-the-u-s-in-q1.html.

Peters, B. 2020. "What to Expect From a Head Transplant." https://www.verywellhealth.com/head-transplant-4801452.

Pultarova, T. 2017. "Why Human Head Transplants Will Never Work." https://www.livescience.com/60987-human-head-transplants-will-never-work.html.

Rapp, N. 2017. "Here's What Every Organ in the Body Would Cost to Transplant." https://fortune.com/2017/09/14/organ-transplant-cost/#:-:text=It's another thing to consider, transplant runs just over %24400%2C000.

Reber, P. 2010. "What is the Memory Capacity of the Human Brain." https://www.scientificamerican.com/article/what-is-the-memory-capacity.

Regalado, A. 2018. "Researchers are keeping pig brains alive outside the body." https://www.technologyreview.co/2018/04/25/240742/researchers-are-keeping-pig-brains-alive-outside-the-body.

Rettner, R. 2014. "Life After Brain Death: Is the Body Still Alive?" *Live Science*.

Sachdeva, K. n.d. "11 Fun Facts About Your Brain." https://www.nm.org/healthbeat/healthy-tips/11-fun-facts-about-your-brain.

Santos-Longhurst, A. 2019. "Does Alcohol Kill Brain Cells?" https://www.healthline/does-alcohol-kill-cells#brain-development.

Sarich, C. n.d. "The Mind vs, Brain Debate (What is Consciousness?)" https://www.cuyamungueinstitute.com/article-and-news/the-mind-vs-brain-debate-what-isconsciousness.

Satsaugi, A. 2011. "What is the difference between the mind and the brain?" https://wwww.researchgate.net/post/What_is_difference_between_mind_and_brain/4e737ebeffea752956000001/citation/download.

Schmid, D. 2018. "Does light [or sound] travel forever?" https://van.physics.illinois.edu/qa/listing.php?id=21368&t=does-light-travel-forever#:-:text=First%2C let's think about why,water%2Cwood%2Cetc).&t.

Schofield, G. 2014. "When does a human being die?" *QJM: An International Journal of Medicine* 108: 605–609. https://doi.org/10.1093/qjmed/hcu239.

Scott, E. "What Is Stress?" Last modified on August 3, 2020. https://www.verywellmind.com/stress-and-health-3145086.

Shah, P. 2020. "Informed Consent." *Stat Pearls – NCBI.* https://www.ncbi.nlm-nih.gov/books/NBK430827.

Shermer, M. 2016. "Radical Life Extension Is Not Around the Corner." https://www.scientificamerican.com/article/radical-life-extension-is-not-around-the-corner.

Smith, S. 2010. "What is the Memory Capacity of the Human Brain?" https://www.cnsnevada.com/what-is-the-memory-capacity-of-a-human-brain/#::text=As a number%2C a "petabyte,2.5 million gigabytes digital memory.

Suskin, Z. 2018. "Body–to-head transplant; a 'caputal' crime? Examining the corpus of ethical and legal issues." *Philosophy, Ethics, and Humanities in Medicine.* https://link.springer.com/article/10.1186/s13010-018-0063-2.

Takahashi, P. n.d. "Healthy Aging. Your Cardiovascular System." Mayo Clinic, Rochester, Minn.

Taylor, G. 2017. "Scientist thinks the world's first 200-year-old person has already been born." https://norwaytoday.info/everyday/scientist-thinks-worlds-first-200-year-old-person-already-born.

Taylor, A. 2017. "Seven body organs you can live without." *The Conversation.*

Than, K. 2006. "The Ethical Dilemmas of Immortality." https://www.livescience.com/10465-ethical-dilemmas-immortality.html.

Thomas, J. 2020. "Can we put a human brain into a robotic body in 100 years from now?" Quora.

Tracey, K. 2020. "Vagus Nerve Stimulation Reduces Inflammation and the Systems of Arthritis." https://www.cesultra.com/blog/vagus-nerve-stimulation-reduces-inflammation-systms-arthritis-part-1/?gclid=EAlalQobChM19tWPOD r6lVQ77Ach.

Tyson, A. 2016. "Use of brain implants in humans." https://doi.org/10.1036/1097-8542.YB160501.

Tyson, P. 2010. "The Future of Brain Transplants." https://www.pbs.org/wghb/nova/article/brain-transplants.

Ungerleider, N. "Not Science Fiction: A Brain In A Box to Let People Live on After Death." https://www.fastcompany.com/3015553/not-science-fiction-a-brain-in-a-box-to-let-people-live-on-after-death.

Villarosal, L. 2003. "How Much Of the Body Is Replaceable?" https://www.nytimes.com/2003/11/11/science/how-much-of-the-body-is-replaceable.html.

Waltz, E. 2020. "How Do Neural Implants Work?" https://spectrum. ieee.org/the-human-os/biomedical/devices/what-is-neural-implant-neuromodulation-brain-implants-electroceuticals-neuralink-definitio.

Williams, J. n.d. "Here Comes the Bionic Man: Disabled People Will Benefit." www.atechnews.com/newsanalysis/bionicman.html.

Wood, D. 2020. "The Five Senses & Their Functions." https://www.study. com/academy/lesson/the-five-senses-their-functions.html.

Youell, J. 2021. "The 25 Most Dangerous Drugs May Not Be What You Think." https://www.therecoveryvillage.com/drug-addiction.

Printed in the United States
by Baker & Taylor Publisher Services